MW01122983

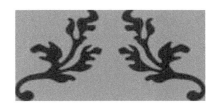

EAT STOP EAT

*Lose Weight, Stay Healthy With The Simple Secret
Of Intermittent Fasting*

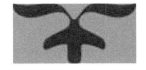

Disclaimer

All erudition supplied in this book is specified for educational and academic purposes only. The author is not in any way in charge of any outcomes that emerge from utilizing this book. Constructive efforts have been made to render information that is both precise and effective; however, the author is not to be held answerable for the accuracy or use/misuse of this information.

Foreword

I will like to thank you for taking the very first step of trusting me and deciding to purchase/read this life-transforming book. Thanks for investing your time and resources on this product.

I can assure you of precise outcomes if you will diligently follow the specific blueprint I lay bare in the information handbook you are currently checking out. It has transformed lives, and I strongly believe it will equally transform your own life too.

All the information I provided in this Do It Yourself piece is easy to absorb and practice.

Table of Contents

INTRODUCTION

Thanks for getting this book and congratulations for taking the decision. The chapters of this book are created to review whatever you need to understand to get going with intermittent fasting. It is a fantastic diet regimen strategy that focuses more on the appropriate time to eat foods instead of the actual food you are consuming. When it comes to utilizing the periodic fast so you will certainly have the capacity to make it work for your method of life, there is a broad range of alternatives.

This overview will provide you with all the information that you require to start with intermittent fasting. We will certainly have a look at what this fast is all about, its wellness benefits, how to eat on this diet method, as well as lots more.

We will also react to some typical worries concerning fasting to make sure that you are entirely prepared to start.

The periodic fast can be an exceptional alternative for those that have actually had trouble losing weight in the past and who now desire something that will work well for them. Ensure to examine this handbook to help you in starting with intermittent fasting today.

There is a great deal of publications on this subject in the marketplace, so thanks once again for picking this one. Every initiative was made to ensure it is jam-packed with useful info, so please find pleasure in it!

CHAPTER ONE
What Is Intermittent Fasting

Now that we have looked at how the American diet is making us unhealthy, let's study an eating design that will make it much easier to lose weight and make you healthier. This section of the book will discuss everything about intermittent fasting, so you can comprehend how it might work for you.

Intermittent fasting includes a dieter cycling between periods where they are permitted to eat and periods where they are expected to fast. This kind of diet doesn't always say which foods you can eat but specifies when you ought to eat. If you desire to reduce weight or get much better health, it is much better to eat healthy foods that benefit you. However, intermittent fasting does not tell you which foods you can and cannot have.

What is intermittent fasting (IF)?

Intermittent Fasting involves restricting the consumption of food for a set period and does not consist of any modifications to the real foods you are eating. Intermittent fasting may be regarded as a natural eating pattern that people are trying to implement and it traces back to our Palaeolithic hunter-gatherer ancestors. The present model of an organised program of intermittent fasting might assist in improving aspects of our health from body composition to longevity and aging.

Intermittent fasting for novices has two rules to follow: (1) Fasting needs to be satisfying and NOT tricky.

 (2) Fasting needs to be easy and not rigid.

From an experienced point of view, I have some tips for intermittent fasting novices. There are two significant reasons for individuals who desire to do Intermittent Fasting (IF) - weight loss or health benefits or both. In any case, it's great to observe these two solutions:

More rules = highly complicated = low chance of success

Fewer rules = less complicated = high opportunity of success

In regards to health, a 24-hour duration without consuming is beneficial because it helps you minimize calories without surrendering what you like to eat on your non-fasting days. More importantly, it stimulates your body to produce more development hormonal agent. Yes, that's right, development hormonal agent, the same one you hear about that the stars require to 'remain young'. Growth hormonal agent has lots of anti-aging advantages, with the most intriguing being fat burning!

There are different forms of intermittent fasting methods; however, all of them split up your days or weeks into consuming periods and fasting periods. What you may be shocked to understand is that the majority of us already fast each day when we are sleeping. You might extend the natural fast time for a bit longer. For example, you may choose to skip breakfast and have your very first meal at midday and your last meal at 8 pm. This would be considered a kind of intermittent fasting.

With this method, you technically fast for sixteen hours every day and after that eat during an eight-hour duration. This form of fasting, likewise called the 16/8 method, is among the popular choices when it pertains to intermittent fasting.

In spite of what you might believe right now, intermittent fasting is simpler than you think. It doesn't take much preparation, and countless individuals who have gone on this diet plan report that they feel much better and have more energy when they are on a fast. At the start, you might struggle a bit with appetite; but it won't take long before your body adapts and gets used to it.

The main thing to bear in mind is that when you

remain in the fasting duration, you are not permitted to eat. However, you may still drink beverages to keep you hydrated.

A few of the choices include tea, coffee, water, and other non-caloric beverages. Some kinds of this fast will enable a little bit of food throughout the fasting periods, but a lot do not. And if you like, it is generally great to take a supplement while you are on this fasting, as long as it does not consist of calories.

Why Fast?

The next question that you might have is why you need to consider fasting in the first place. Human beings have been going through a period of fasting for several years. Sometimes they did this as a necessity because they were unable to discover any food to eat. There were also moments that the fasting was done for spiritual reasons.

Religious beliefs such as Christianity, Islam, and Buddhism mandate some varieties of fasting. It is also natural to fast when you are feeling sick.

Although fasting often has a negative undertone, there is nothing abnormal about fasting. In truth, our bodies are well geared up to deal with times when we need to go without eating. Numerous procedures within the body system alter when we go on a fast. This enables our bodies to continue functioning during periods of scarcity.

When we fast, we get a substantial reduction in insulin and blood in addition to an extreme boost in what is referred to as human growth hormonal agent. While this was something that was initially done for a limited few, it is now used to help people to lose weight. With fasting, burning fat becomes simpler, much more comfortable, and efficient.

Some people decide to go on a fast because it can help their metabolic process. This type of fasting is right for improving different health disorders and illnesses.

There is likewise some evidence that demonstrates

how intermittent fasting can assist you in living longer. Studies reveal that rodents can extend their life expectancy with intermittent fasting.

Other research reveals that fasting can provide protection against numerous illnesses such as Alzheimer's, cancer, type-2 diabetes, and heart disease. And then there are some who choose to go on an intermittent fast for a hassle-free lifestyle. Fasting can be an efficient life hack. For instance, the fewer meals you have to make, the simpler your life will be.

How does intermittent fasting work?

Intermittent fasting is the technique of scheduling your meals for your body to obtain the most out of them. Instead of reducing your calorie usage in half, denying yourself of all the foods you love, or diving into a classy diet plan trend, intermittent fasting is a natural, rational, and healthy and balanced technique of eating that advances weight loss. There are several ways to approach intermittent fasting.

It's specified as a particular eating pattern. This technique concentrates on changing when you take in, as opposed to what you consume.

When you begin intermittent fasting, you will more than likely maintain your calories.

Intake is also the same, however, as opposed to spreading your meals throughout the day, you will certainly eat larger dishes throughout a shorter amount of time. Instead of eating 3 to 4 meals a day, you might consume one large meal at 11 am, after that an additional big meal at 6 pm, without any meal in between 11 am and 6 pm, and also after 6 pm, no meal up until 11 am the following day. This is just one strategy of recurring fasting, the others will be described in this book in later phases.

You must first comprehend why this strategy functions. Intermittent fasting is a method utilised by lots of bodybuilders, professional athletes, and physical fitness masters to keep their muscle high and their body fat low. It is a primary method that allows you to eat the foods you take pleasure in, while still encouraging fat loss and muscle gain or upkeep. Intermittent fasting can be done short term or long term, but the very best outcomes originate from adopting this approach into your daily lifestyle.

The word "fasting" may worry the average person; intermittent fasting does not relate to starving yourself. To comprehend the principals behind successful intermittent fasting, we'll initially review the body's digestion state: the fed state and the fasting state.

For 3 to 5 hours after eating, your body is in what is referred to as the "fed state." Throughout the fed state, your insulin levels increase to soak up and digest your meal. When your insulin levels are high, your body will find it difficult to burn fat.

Insulin is a hormone given by the pancreas to manage glucose levels in the bloodstream. Its purpose is to control; insulin is technically a storage hormonal agent. When insulin levels become so high, your body starts burning your food for energy rather than your saved fat which is why increased levels of it prevent weight loss.

After the 3 to 5 hours are up, your body has completed the meal processing, and you enter the post-absorptive state. The post-absorptive state lasts from 8 to 12 hours. When your body gets in after this time space is the fasted state. Because your body has completely processed your food by this point, your insulin levels are reduced, making your stored fat available for shedding.

In the abstained state, your body has no diet to use for power, so your conserved fat is melted instead. Recurring fasting enables your body to reach a sophisticated weight loss state that you would typically get to with the average three square meals daily eating pattern. This aspect alone is the reason many individuals observe fast outcomes with intermittent fasting without also making alterations to their workout routines, the quantity they consume, or what they consume. They are simply altering the timing as well as pattern of their food intake. It might take some time to get when you begin an intermittent fasting program but don't get discouraged! Simply get back into your program if you slip up when you can. Avoid beating yourself up, or feeling guilty. Negative self-talk will only lengthen your return to your program.

Making a lifestyle change involves a deliberate effort, and nobody expects you to do it entirely right now. If you are not used to fasting (without eating), intermittent fasting will take some getting used to. As long as you select the right technique for you, remain focused, and stay focused, you will master it in no time.

Unlike some of the other diet plan that you may undertake, the intermittent fast will work better. It uses your body and how it works to its advantage in helping you to lose weight. When you first hear about it, it is easy to get a bit afraid about fasting. You might assume that you need to spend weeks and days without eating (and who has the self-control to quit their food for that long even when they do want to reduce weight?) and that it will be too tough for you.

Intermittent fasting is a bit varied than you may think. Not just is it tough not to eat for weeks at a time but it is also not good for the body. If you end up doing the fast for too long, your body will frequently go into starvation mode. because it assumes that you are experiencing food scarcity.

Then the body will work on conserving the calories and assisting you to hold on to the fat and calories for as long as possible. This suggests that not only are you hungry, but you are likewise missing out on slimming down.

You don't have to think too much about how this intermittent fast will work in the hunger mode. The intermittent fast is efficient because you are not going to fast for so long that the body enters into this starvation mode and stops reducing weight. Rather, it will make the fast persist long enough that you will be able to speed up the metabolic process.

With the intermittent fast, you will discover that when you opt for a couple of hours without eating (normally no more than 2 - 4 hours), the body is not going to go right into starvation mode. Instead, it is going to consume the calories that are readily available. If you eat the right quantity of calories for the day, the body is going to revert to making use of the stored reserves of fat and use it as energy. As such, when following an intermittent fasting plan, you subject your body to burn more fat without putting in additional work.

Here are a few fasting suggestions for success:

Primarily, it is essential not to expect to see results from your new way of life immediately. Instead, you need to focus on devoting a minimum of 30 days to the process before you can start to judge the outcomes precisely.

Secondly, it is vital to remember that the high quality of food you place into your body still matters as it will simply take a few fast food meals to reverse all of your hard job.

For the ideal outcomes, you should include a light exercise regimen during fasting days as well as a much more basic routine for full-calorie days.

Intermittent Fasting refers to nutritional consuming patterns that include not consuming or restricting calories for a long term period.

Periodic Fasting (There are different subgroups of periodic fasting each with individual variation in the period of the fast; some for hours, others for days). This has ended up being an extremely preferred topic in the scientific research community as a result of the prospective benefits on physical fitness as well as wellness that are being discovered.

How The Process Works

The diet you follow whilst intermittent fasting will be determined by the results that you are searching for and where you are starting from. So take a look at yourself and ask the question, "What do I desire from this?"

If you are seeking to lose a significant amount of weight, then you are going to have to look at your diet plan more closely, but if you want to lose a few pounds for the beach, then you might find that a couple weeks of intermittent fasting can do that for you.

There are many different ways you can do intermittent fasting, we are just going to look at the 24-hour fasting system which is what I used to lose 27 pounds over a 2-month duration. You might feel some hunger pangs, but these will pass, and as you end up being more accustomed to intermittent fasting, you might find as I have that feeling of hunger no longer present you with an issue.

While fasting, it is advisable to drink plenty of water to avoid dehydration. Tea and coffee are okay as long as you take a splash of milk. If you are worried that you are not getting sufficient nutrients into your body, then you may consider a juice made from celery, broccoli, ginger, and lime, which will taste fantastic and get some abundant nutrient liquid into your body. If you can handle it, then it would be best to stick to the coffee, water, and tea.

Whatever your diet plan is whether it's healthy or not, you ought to see weight reduction after about three weeks of intermittent fasting. However, do not be dissuaded if you don't discover much development initially. It's not a race and it's much better to drop weight in a direct style over time rather than crash-losing a few pounds which you will put straight back on. After the first month, you may wish to have a look at your diet on non-fasting days and eliminate high sugar foods and any junk that you usually consume. I have found that intermittent fasting over the long term tends to make me eager to consume more healthy foods as a natural routine.

If you are practising intermittent fasting for bodybuilding then you may wish to consider taking a look at your macro-nutrients and understanding just how much protein and carbohydrate you require to consume. This is much more complex, and you can discover information about this on several sites which you will need to investigate for the best outcomes.

There are lots of advantages to intermittent fasting, which you will see as you progress. A few of these advantages consist of more energy, less bloating, a clearer mind, and a general sensation of wellness. It's crucial not to succumb to any temptation to binge eat after a fasting duration, as this will negate the impact gained from the intermittent fasting period.

So in conclusion, just by following a twice a week 24-hour intermittent fasting strategy for a few weeks, you will slim down. However, if you can enhance your diet plan on the days that you do not fast then you will lose more weight. And if you can stay with this system, then you will keep the weight off without turning to any fad diet or diet plans that are difficult to adhere to.

Intermittent Fasting As An Alternative To Traditional Exercise

In this part of the book, we will use the concept of intermittent fasting as an option for conventional exercise for weight-loss. As we will see in this discussion, the two are not so different and can be an excellent method to accelerate the impacts of weight loss.

As opposed to exercising, which needs physical exertion, intermittent fasting is merely a way of weight reduction that needs you to avoid eating for a short amount of time. Once or twice a week, the duration of these fasts usually lasts around 24 hours.

A massive plus for utilising intermittent fasting rather than regular exercise is the capability to reduce weight without having to hit the fitness centre. This can save you a bunch of time; specifically, if you lead a hectic life and can't spare the time, you won't need to do exercise.

It likewise indicates that with this technique, diet ends up being a significant determinant in your weight-loss progress. I generally state that diet and nutrition need to be doing eighty to ninety percent of the work on your fat loss program. You need not to ever count on a workout routine solely for lasting weight loss. This holds true, since diet is a significant controller of blood hormone levels, and those hormones that affect weight reduction are necessary if you desire to lose fat.

Intermittent Fasting Compared To Exercise

In a traditional fat loss routine, you would want to produce a calorie deficit. You can do this by diet or exercise alone, or you can integrate the two.

When you exercise, blood hormone levels of insulin drops. You also see that the human growth hormonal agent (HGH) hormone levels increase if your work out is extreme. These conditions are required for fat loss to occur.

It has been studied and revealed to be real that by fasting for merely 24 hours, you can create the same hormonal agent blood levels that workout does. If you merely fasted as soon as or two times a week for approximately 24 hours, you might recreate the impacts that exercise does without having to workout at all.

This is good news for those that dislike to work out or don't have adequate time for it.

A crucial thing to bear in mind is my suggestion that you use a combination of the two for the most optimum results. They will work separately; but you can get outcomes much quicker with this course of action. Hope this helps increase your understanding of intermittent fastin

CHAPTER TWO
Benefits of Intermittent Fasting

Recurring fasting is an increasingly popular weight-loss choice as well as a wellness monitoring device. It has numerous essential advantages over various other strategies. Here are five of them.

1: Counting calories is not needed in periodic fasting. Practically all nutritional methods consist of counting calories.

2: You do not need to deprive yourself in intermittent fasting. Fasting is not consuming, and when you stop the fast, you can eat if you are hungry.

3: Your body does not attempt to hang on to its fat stores when recurring fasting. When you can eat to your satisfaction, as holds true on a fasting diet strategy, your body reacts by using up your body fat.

4: An intermittent fasting diet plan is less restrictive than other diets. It is entirely possible and also even useful to have some flexibility in what you consume.

5: An intermittent fasting diet plan adapts to you. This is the genuine charm of this approach. Rather than trying to locate exactly the best variety of grams of carbs or everything at 10 am, you fit your day-to-day fast to your life and goals. Some find a 16 hour fast from evening till the following day at lunch break functions most excellently. Others choose a 24-hour cycle or perhaps a 4-hour consuming home window. All of these are feasible as well as have various benefits. It is a way of living as opposed to a diet regimen plan.

Results You Can Expect From Intermittent Fasting

Intermittent fasting is a feeding pattern that rotates in between periods of fasting and managed eating. Among the recurring fasting strategies is alternate-day fasting, where you can take a routine diet regimen strategy on specific days of the week and also fast on some.

The other fasting kind is wherein consuming is limited to a specific time home window within a day. This suggests restricting consuming within an 8-hour home window consuming duration, which implies an individual consumes every 8 hours. Some individuals nonetheless decrease the period to either 6, 4, and even two hours according to their benefit. The lengthiest time that a person can remain without food on intermittent fasting is 36 hrs. If practiced properly, it can lead to several positive health effects.

For situations, intermittent fasting advertises general health and wellness. Intermittent fasting will, for that reason, guard the body from diseases.

Periodic fasting causes enhanced mind wellness. The continued breakdown of body fats allows the liver to produce ketone bodies if the fasting continues for some time.

This sort of fasting, furthermore, improves body physical conditioning and loss of weight. Integrated fasting and workout raise the effects of drivers as well as cellular elements to make sure that the breakdown of glycogen and also fats is optimized. Working out while hungry, for that reason, forces the body to burn saved fats for considerable weight-loss.

The program is also recognized to protect against cognitive decline. The research was accomplished in 2006 on laboratory mice, in which water maze examinations were used to review cognitive functions of lab mice on a regular diet plan as well as those on intermittent fasting. It was discovered that mice placed on intermittent fasting experienced slower cognitive declines. Intermittent fasting will also enhance muscle mass building, especially in men. The body makes use of maintained body fats to sustain the exercises if training is done while fasting.

Intermittent fasting is a healthy and balanced method, but it may lead to anxiety in individuals that can not sufficiently sustain it. It calls for dedication and decision to move with the adjustments in diet because only consistency will certainly achieve these favorable results.

CHAPTER THREE
Types of Intermittent Fasting

There are a few significant kinds of intermittent fasting that you can choose to work with. These fasts can all work, and the one that's right for you will depend upon your personal choices, schedule, and way of life. A few of the fasting alternatives that you can go with include:

The 16/8 technique: This one will ask you to fast for 16 hours each day and eat during the other 8 hours. So, you may choose to just consume from midday to 8 pm or from 10 am to 6 pm. You can select whichever eight-hour window that you like.

Eat-Stop-Eat: Once or two times every week, you will not eat anything from supper until dinner the next day. This provides you with a 24-hour fast but still allows you to eat on each of the days that you are fasting.

The 5:2 diet plan: You will choose 2 days of the week without eating. During those two days, you are only allowed to have up to 500-600 calories each day.

Though there are variations of the three that are listed above, some individuals can decide to restrict their windows a lot more and only eat for 4 hours and fast for about twenty on this diet plan. A lot of people who go on these fasts do so because it's the most convenient to stick with. If you choose to go with the 16/8 method, it will offer you some terrific lead to the procedure.

Periodic fasting is reputable and basic. It helps you limit the amount of calories that you are taking in and sheds much more fat as well as calories than you would with a traditional diet plan.

It comes in different forms and each may have a detailed set of special advantages. The most popular intermittent fasting programs are alternating day fasting, time-restricted feeding, as well as customized fasting.

1. Alternate Day Fasting:

This technique includes alternating days of absolutely

no calories (from food or beverage) with days of free feeding and eating whatever you desire.

This plan has been revealed to assist with weight reduction, improve blood cholesterol and triglyceride (fat) levels, and improve markers for inflammation in the blood.

Because of the reported hunger during fasting days, the primary downfall with this type of intermittent fasting is that it is the most difficult to stick with.

2. Customized Fasting - 5:2 diet

Customized fasting is a protocol with configured fasting days, but the fasting days do permit for some food consumption. Typically 20-25% of regular calories are allowed to be taken in on fasting days, so if you usually consume 2000 calories on routine eating days, you would be allowed 400-500 calories on fasting days.

This procedure is excellent for weight loss, body composition, and might likewise benefit the policy of blood sugar level, lipids, and inflammation. Studies have shown the 5:2 technique to be useful for weight loss, improve/lower inflammation markers in the blood, and show signs of trending improvements in insulin resistance. In animal research studies, this changed fasting 5:2 diet plan led to decreased fat, lowered cravings hormones (leptin), and boosted levels of a healthy protein responsible for renovations in fat loss as well as blood sugar guideline (adiponectin).

The changed 5:2 fasting method is very easy to comply with and has some negative unfavorable results which consists of hunger, low energy, and also some inflammation when beginning the program. As opposed to this nevertheless, studies have actually kept in mind improvements such as lowered stress, less rage, much less fatigue, enhancements in self-confidence, and an extra desirable mindset.

3. Time-restricted Feeding:.

If you understand anybody that has stated they are doing recurring fasting, chances are it is in the kind of time-restricted feeding. Daily fasting periods in time-restricted feeding may range from 12-20 hrs, with the most common method being 16/8 (no eating for 16 hrs, eating calories for 8). On a 16/8 time-restricted eating program someone may consume their initial meal at 7AM as well as last meal at 3PM (fast from 3PM-7AM), while another individual might eat their first dish at 1PM and last meal at 9PM (fast from 9PM-1PM).

Time-Restricted eating is one of the simplest strategies of intermittent fasting. Time-restricted feeding is a superb program to comply with for weight-loss and also body framework enhancements in addition to other general wellness advantages. From animal research studies, time restricted feeding guards against weight problems, high insulin levels, fatty liver disease, and swelling.

The easy application and appealing outcomes of time-restricted feeding could potentially make it an excellent option for weight-loss and chronic illness prevention/management. When executing this procedure, it may be useful to begin with a lower fasting-to-eating ratio like 12/12 hours and ultimately work your method to as much as 16/8 hours.

CHAPTER FOUR
Effects Of Intermittent Fasting On Weight Loss

Food craving is the unchecked want for eating brought upon by outdoors forces; this takes place in times of battle and deficiency when food is limited. Food is readily offered, nevertheless, we choose not to eat it as a result of spiritual, health and wellness, or other elements.

Fasting is as old as mankind, much older than any other kinds of diet regimens. Ancient people, like the Greeks, recognized that there was something naturally sensible to routine fasting.

Before the introduction of farming, people did not eat three dishes a day plus snacking in between. When we found food which may be days or humans resources apart, we took in just what we needed. From a development point of view, taking in three meals a day is not needed for survival. Or else, we would not have in reality endured as a specie.

Fasting is actually poor for service! Food manufacturers advise us to eat as many dishes as we can in a day.

Fasting has no main period. It could be done for a few hours to several days to months on end. Recurring fasting is an eating pattern where we cycle between fasting as well as routine eating.

Fasting has been engaged in by millions and countless people for countless years. Countless studies have actually exposed that it has massive wellness benefits.

What Happens When We Eat Constantly?

Prior to becoming part of the benefits of periodic fasting, it is best to comprehend why eating 5-6 dishes a day or every couple of hours (the exact opposite of fasting) may do even more harm than good.

When we eat, we ingest food energy. Fat causes a smaller sized insulin effect, however fat is barely ever consumed alone.

Insulin has two major functions -

It permits the body to start making use of food energy promptly. Insulin takes glucose right into the body cells to be used as energy. Healthy and balanced healthy proteins do not necessarily elevate blood glucose yet it can promote insulin.

When the restriction is gotten to, the liver starts changing sugar right into fat. The fat is afterwards done away with in the liver (also, it finishes up being fatty liver) or stored in the body (regularly kept as persistent or natural persistent stomach fat).

When we eat as well as snack throughout the day, we are continuously in a fed state and our insulin degrees stay high. Basically, we could be investing a great deal of the day maintaining our food energy.

What Should Be Expected From Intermittent Fasting

Intermittent Fasting is an eating pattern that substitutes between durations of fasting and also managed eating. It is an all-natural dietary technique divided right into many types. Amongst the intermittent fasting approaches is alternate-day fasting, where a person takes a normal diet regimen on certain days of the week as well as fasts on some. During the fasting days, one does not avoid food, yet, rather lowers calorie consumption to 1/4 of the normal diet plan.

The other fasting type of eating is restricted to a certain time home window within a day. The lengthiest time that a person can remain without food on intermittent fasting is 36 hrs.

For conditions, intermittent fasting advertises basic health. It significantly reduces yearnings for junk food and also sugars. The technique normalizes insulin in addition to the leptin degree of level of sensitivity. Insulin resistance adds to health problems such as diabetes mellitus, cancer and also heart infections. Intermittent fasting will, therefore, guard the body from such diseases.

Periodic fasting causes enhanced mind wellness. The continued breakdown of body fats causes the liver to create ketone bodies if the not eating continues for some time.

This kind of fasting furthermore enhances body fitness and also loss of weight. Integrated fasting as well as workout increases mobility so that the breakdown of glycogen as well as fats is optimized. Exercising while hungry, for that reason, forces the body to melt saved fats for substantial weight-loss.

The program is furthermore understood to avoid cognitive decrease. The research was executed in 2006 on lab mice, in which water puzzle tests were utilized to evaluate cognitive features of lab mice on a regular diet plan as well as those on recurring fasting. It was found that mice placed on intermittent fasting experienced slower cognitive decreases, which also applies to humans.

Recurring fasting will additionally increase muscle building, particularly in men. If training is done while fasting, the body uses maintained body fats to maintain the workouts.

Finally, recurring fasting is a healthy practice, however it may result in anxiety in individuals who cannot appropriately sustain it. Since consistency will give positive results, it needs commitment and also resolution.

Two myths that pertain to intermittent fasting.

Myths 1 - You Must Eat Three Meals Per Day: This "rule" that is typical in Western society was not developed based on the proof for enhanced health, but was embraced as the typical pattern for settlers and eventually ended up being the norm. There exists a lack of scientific reasoning justifying the three meal-a-day practice as recent research studies may be showing that less meals and more fasting are ideal for human health. A research study also revealed that a single meal a day with the same quantity of daily calories is much better for weight reduction and body composition than three meals each day. Intermittent fasting allows a person to best eat 1-2 meals per day. This finding is a fundamental concept that is theorised into intermittent fasting and those opting to do it.

Myth 2 - You Need Breakfast, It's the Most Important Meal of The Day: Many false cases about the outright demand for an everyday morning meal have actually been made. The most regular insurance claims being "morning meal increases your metabolic procedure" as well as "morning meal lowers food consumption later on in the day".

CHAPTER FIVE
Why You Should Try Intermittent Fasting

There is an excellent choice of various diet plans that you can pick from. Some help you limit your carb intake and focus on the healthy fats and proteins. Some will restrict your fat consumption and also concentrate on healthy, balanced and superb carbs.

With all of the alternatives in the industry, and with at least a few of them being reputable selections for lowering weight, you might wonder why you must choose intermittent fasting. This phase will look at the various benefits of periodic fasting and also how it will make a distinction in your health.

Change the feature of cells, hormones, and genetics

Numerous things take place in your body when you do not eat for some time. Your body will start initiating procedures for cell repair work as well as altering some of your hormonal agent degrees, which makes maintained body fat easily accessible

Other adjustments that can occur in the body include: Insulin degrees. Your insulin degrees will come by a reasonable bit, which makes it easier for the body to melt fat

Human development hormone agent: The blood levels of the development hormonal agent can significantly rise. Greater levels of this hormonal representative can assist in the construction of muscular tissue as well as burn fat.

Mobile repair work: The body will certainly begin important mobile repair procedures, such as getting rid of all the waste from cells.

Gene expression: Some helpful modifications happen in countless genetics that will help you to live longer and also guard against disease.

Drop weight and body fat.

Lots of people go on an intermittent quick to lose

weight. Essentially, intermittent fasting will naturally help you in consuming fewer meals. You will certainly wind up absorbing less calories, which will result in weight reduction.

Fasting improves the hormone feature to assist with weight-loss.

Greater development hormone levels as well as reduced insulin assist your body to breakdown fat as well as utilize it for energy. This is why short-term fasting can boost your metabolic process by a minimum of three percent.

On one hand, it enhances your metabolic rate to ensure that you burn a whole lot extra calories while also minimizing just how much you eat. According to a 2014 evaluation of specialist research study on intermittent fasting, people could lose up to 8 percent of their body weight in less than 24 weeks.

Helps with diabetes

Type-2 diabetes is an illness that has increased in

current decades. Anything that minimizes your insulin resistance needs to help decrease your blood glucose levels and also guard you against type 2 diabetes mellitus. Some researches show exactly how.

Periodic fasting can be beneficial to insulin resistance and also help create an amazing reduction in blood glucose levels.

In several research studies on intermittent fasting, blood glucose was lowered by three to six percent, while insulin level was reduced by twenty to thirty-one percent. One research study on diabetic rats also revealed that periodic fasting might secure the rat against kidney damages, which is a typical issue with more extreme kinds of diabetes. This reveals that recurring fasting could be an outstanding option for anyone with a higher risk of getting type-2 diabetic issues.

There are some differences between the genders. There is one research that disclosed that for females, blood glucose level control might worsen after undergoing the periodic fast for a couple of weeks. Before you start, it is best to talk to your doctor about your diet plan.

Streamlines life

While this may not be considered a wellness advantage like the others, it is still a crucial one to point out. Most individuals discover that intermittent fasting can make their lives less complex. They figure out that they do not have to focus way too much on the calories they are eating, as long as they remain within the hours that they are allowed to eat. They can go a few days a week without having to fret about making a meal. Generally, this diet regimen plan can make your life less complicated.

When you can eliminate a few of the job that you are required to do throughout the day and emphasize on another thing, you can end up with less stress and anxiety in your life. All of us understand the negative impact extreme stress can have on our wellness and life. When you can reduce stress, it is a lot simpler to be the healthiest variation of yourself.

Great for the heart

Heart disease is among the most significant diseases worldwide.

Periodic Fasting can aid with a few of these threat facets, such as decreasing blood sugar levels, inflammatory markers, blood triglycerides, cholesterol as well as high blood stress.

The most considerable issue is that a lot of research studies on intermittent fasting has in fact been done on animals. We need to have even more studies that evaluate intermittent fasting as well as heart health in human beings.

Can aid with cancer

Several individuals have cancer cells yearly. The unchecked advancement of cells defines this horrible condition. Fasting has been disclosed to have some outstanding benefits when it pertains to your metabolic process, which may cause a lowered threat of cancer cells.

Some human research studies disclose that individuals with cancer cells who fasted could lessen a few of the side effects that include chemotherapy.

Useful for the mind

What is depicted as fantastic for the body also benefits the mind. Intermittent fasting can help improve metabolic functions that are understood to aid the mind to stay healthy. This could include assisting with insulin resistance, blood sugar level decrease, lowered inflammation and oxidative tension.

There have actually been several research studies done on rats that demonstrate just how intermittent fasting can boost the development of brand-new afferent nerve cells, which improves the mind's function. Not eating can likewise assist in boosting the sections of the brain deprived of neurotrophic aspect. When the brain is lacking in this, it can activate depression together with a few other mind worries.

Assists with cellular fixing

The cells in the body can start a waste removal which is a quick process recognized as autophagy that involves the cells breaking down and metabolizing any kind of healthy proteins that cannot be made use of any longer. With an

increased amount of autophagy, it might help guard the body against diseases such as Alzheimer's and also cancer cells.

May prevent Alzheimer

Alzheimer is amongst the most common neurodegenerative illness. There is no cure for Alzheimer's, so the best step is to prevent it from happening as much as possible. One study that was carried out on rats showed that intermittent fasting could be able to delay the start of Alzheimer illness or minimize the intensity of it.

Some reports have really shown that a way of life modification that included some daily, or a minimum of regular, temporary fasts aided to improve the signs of Alzheimer's in 9 out of 10 clients. Pet research studies additionally reveal that this kind of fasting may aid in safeguarding against various other neurodegenerative diseases, such as Huntington's illness and Parkinson's.

Intermittent fasting is a pattern, and research studies on ways it makes your body healthier is still brand-new. It will require some time to examine all the advantages of recurring fasting.

Intermittent Fasting can help you in living much longer.

Amongst one of the most interesting attributes of periodic fasting is that it can assist you live longer. There have actually been several research studies of rats that demonstrated exactly how.

Intermittent fasting may help prolong their life-span - comparable to what takes place when you place a constant calorie limitation. In some of the research studies, the impacts were amazing. In one of them, when the rats did not eat every other day, they ended up living 83 percent longer than the rats that didn't do fasting.

It has truly been tough to reveal an increase in life-span due to the fact that periodic fasting has yet to be analyzed on people. However, it is still a prominent concept for those who are trying to stop aging. With the recognized benefits to the body's metabolism, it is not uncommon that individuals think that intermittent fasting will certainly able to help them live much longer, healthier lives.

As you can see, there are huge benefits of choosing the repeating fasting diet regimen. Even though we simply reviewed a few of them, there have actually been many research studies done on the effects of this diet plan as well as why it can benefit you. Whether you are attempting to boost brain health, live a lot longer, drop weight, or obtain even more power, periodic fasting can boost your life. It does not have any one of these drawbacks.

CHAPTER SIX
Why Intermittent Fasting is Mainly for Women

For women who have an interest in weight-loss, intermittent fasting may appear like a terrific option, but lots of people would like to know, should females fast? Is intermittent fasting efficient for women? There have been a few fundamental research studies about intermittent fasting, which can help to shed some light on this intriguing brand-new dietary trend.

Intermittent fasting is also called alternate-day fasting, although there are certainly some variations on this diet. *The American Journal of Clinical Nutrition* performed a research study just recently that enrolled 16 obese men and ladies on a 10-week program. On the fasting days, individuals took in food that is 25% of their estimated energy requirements. The rest of the time, they got dietary counselling, and were not given a particular standard to follow throughout this time.

What made this an interesting discovery was that many individuals had to lose more weight than these study participants before seeing the same changes. It was a remarkable find which has spurred a fantastic number of individuals to try fasting.

Intermittent fasting for females has some beneficial effects. Women who are following a healthy diet and workout plan may be struggling with persistent fat, but fasting is a realistic solution to this.

Intermittent Fasting For Women Over 50

Undoubtedly our bodies and our metabolism changes when we strike menopause. One of the most significant changes that women over 50 experience is that they have a slower metabolic process, and they begin to put on weight. Fasting might be an excellent way to prevent this weight and reverse gain. Research studies have shown that this fasting pattern assists in controlling hunger, and people who follow it regularly do not experience the very same cravings that others do. Intermittent fasting can prevent you from consuming too much on an everyday basis if you're over 50 and trying to adjust to your slower metabolic process.

When you reach 50, your body also begins to form some chronic diseases like high cholesterol and high blood pressure. Intermittent fasting has been revealed to reduce both cholesterol and blood pressure, even without a terrific deal of weight reduction. If you've begun to notice your numbers increasing at the hospital each year, you can bring them back down with fasting, even without losing much weight.

Intermittent fasting might not be an excellent concept for every single woman. Anybody with a particular health condition or who tends to be hypoglycemic must consult with a physician. This new dietary pattern has specific benefits for females who naturally store more fat in their bodies and might have a problem getting rid of these fat deposits.

CHAPTER SEVEN
How To Practise Intermittent Fasting Healthily And Safely

Periodic fasting can enhance wellness, reduce the risk of severe disease, and promote longevity. Possibly you're mesmerized and intend to try but don't exactly know how to begin. Or possibly you have actually tried it a couple of times and found it challenging. This brief write-up will give you requirements and methods to practice intermittent fasting safely and also successfully. Please look into the contraindications at the end of this brief write-up before doing a fast.

There are three primary techniques to do intermittent fasting - a) only consume from 6pm to bedtime on a daily basis, b) a 24-hour fast on alternative days, or c) a couple of 36-hour fasts every week. It's worth exploring with all three strategies to see which functions ideally for you in regards to your means of life and the effect on your health. The standards I've offered you below are mostly for the 36hr fasting, but several are useful for the 24hr fast.

Choose a day that isn't busy or taxing since you might experience some detox reactions. Make sure you have the option to take a break if you need to. You will get much more out of the experience if you make time to still your mind, reflect on your strategy, consider, and also pay attention to your internal assistance. Get support from your loved ones before you start. It's superb to fast with your partner so you can both influence each other as well as share experiences.

Eat lightly on the eve of the fasting by choosing a large salad or vegetables with some lean healthy protein. There is no point gorging yourself the evening before due to the fact that it will cause you to feel hungrier while you fast. It's best to also stop alcohol.

Keep your body moisturized throughout the fast as it has an essential requirement for fluid. Have at least 2 liters of liquid throughout the day.

Have 1 or 2 glasses of veggie juice as it will supply crucial electrolytes along with giving you a health-boosting alkalizing outcome. Try juicing celery, cucumber, fennel, watercress, and also chicory. Don't use carrots and beets as they are fairly high in sugar.

Don't battle the starving sensation because you most possibly will. Just be with the experience without judgment, instead of enduring it (however take a look at basic 10 listed here).

Take part in light exercise such as walking, stretching, and also moderate yoga exercise. This is not the moment to do an intense fitness workout or anything too strenuous.

Include some breathing exercises such as yogic pranayama. A couple of minutes of practice offers impressive gain from cleaning to improving energy.

If you usually have lots of caffeine and also sugar in your diet regimen, they can worsen your fast. Instead rest, opt for a walk, and also practice breathing technique workouts.

Listen to your body as well. If you really feel unhealthy or the hunger gets =too much then have some food. Stop the fast gently in the morning. Have water or herb tea and also a piece of fruit when you get up, then 30min later have your typical breakfast. Eat as normal for the rest of the day (you most likely will not really feel the need to eat much).

Take pleasure in the fast and how you really feel after the fast. Be alert to adjustments in your energy, feelings, and also structure of mind. You may observe food is much more satisfying on the day after the fast because your senses are raised.

Recognize that it can take a pair of initiatives to get used to this method. After some weeks, your body will get used to it and the benefits you truly feel will absolutely increase as the discomfort simultaneously lowers.

Contra-Indications

Avoid reoccurring fasting if you are pregnant, diabetic, experiencing a significant illness, or taking any prescribed medications. If doubtful, it is best to consult your physician.

How To Do Intermittent Fasting As a Novice

In a perfect situation, two sessions of 24-hour fasts in a week will certainly be exceptional enough to produce substantial health and also weight reduction advantages. For newbies, you are not expected to start with a 24-hour fast, unless you are sure that you can do it.

Recurring Fasting: There is no fundamental standard of doing it. Just try it as well as make it work for you. Allow simplicity and also versatility be your fasting motto. Do deficient demanding for yourself.

To do intermittent fasting as a newbie, I would specify that you 'clear your mind from other weight-loss methods and concentrate on IF'. This is your preliminary action towards Intermittent Fasting success. If you are establishing your feet onto the route of recurring fasting, it is much better to place these concepts apart at least for the duration you are attempting Intermittent Fasting.

Do you have your IF mindset all set? After that begin with 'miss dish' as well as see how your body reacts. I would certainly specify this as the simplest method to start your intermittent fasting trip.

Pick a day to 'avoid breakfast'. Have fresh juice, water or tea instead. No coffee please. If that work outs fine, try to 'avoid lunch' and proceed slowly. Anybody can do a 24-hour fast with an ideal fasting frame of mind. One beneficial suggestion is not to think about food. Avoid social talk at the cupboard over lunch hour. Take a stroll or do some simple exercises.

You can also discover these Intermittent Fasting choices:

- Condensed consuming window, e.g. consume ONLY in between 11am and 5pm;

- Skip dish on an unanticipated basis, as long as it is natural and does not conflict with your day-to-day job;

- Early and late, i.e. avoid lunch;

- One dish a day, ideally supper simply when you are unwinded and also derive enjoyment from your food.

To continue with it, fasting needs to be enjoyable and not difficult. When you are called upon for company, notify the other person that you are not eating, do not interrupt your job. Do it as you see fit and as well as your routine allows.

CHAPTER EIGHT
How To Engage In Intermittent Fasting

A usual point that many individuals enjoy concerning periodic fasting is the fact that it provides you with a lot of alternatives. As reviewed, there are a couple of ways that you can do an Intermittent Fast based on your schedule and way of life. Some individuals discover that they have a number of hectic days during the week and as a result will certainly fast on those days. Others love the idea of limiting their eating home window and also doing a little fast every day.

The fasting approach that you choose depends on you. Every one of them can be effective and will supply you with a few of the advantages that you are browsing for. Let's consider some fasting options that you can opt for, so you can choose the finest one for you.

The 16/8 Method.

This is one of the most typical approaches that you can

utilize in intermittent fasting. It requires you to fast for about 14 to 16 hrs everyday and eat for the rest of the hours. During this consuming window, you are still able to fit in two to three meals without a concern. This is probably to match the consuming routine that you are used to, nonetheless it still limits you so that you do not eat throughout the day.

This strategy is extra straightforward than you think. It is merely about not eating any type of meals after you are done with dinner and afterwards missing morning meal, or at least having a late morning meal. You are currently not eating for 16 hours if you finish your last dish at 8 at evening and then do not consume anything until lunchtime the next day.

You simply need to be mindful concerning the late-night snacks. If you eat them, you will have to avoid morning meal in the morning.

Some individuals have problems with this since they feel deprived in the morning and feel they need to consume morning meal. You can merely shift the morning meal to later on in the day. If you choose to take breakfast at 10 in the early morning instead of 8 after you quit eating by 6 in the evening, you would still be within the 16-hour home window.

This is the option that you must possibly choose if you're a lady.

Females commonly do well with these much shorter fasts and they might want to consider opting for 14 to 15 hours in between eating given that this is more reliable for them.

Throughout the fast, you are allowed to drink water, tea, coffee, as well as various other beverages that are non-caloric to assist in minimizing the hunger discomforts that occur.

Additionally, you have to try and stick to much healthier foods throughout your consuming home window. It is not an excellent suggestion to consume a great deal of junk food during this moment. Some people like to use a low-carb diet plan when they get on intermittent fast since it aids with food cravings and allows for a lot more better end results.

The 5:2 diet

Another choice that you can select is the 5:2 diet regimen. This set allows you to eat generally for 5 days throughout the week in addition to limiting your intake to no better than 600 calories on each of the other 2 days. This is occasionally called "the Fast Diet strategy".

You can pick any days of the week as your fasting days, as long as you do not have them back to back. Pick your two busiest days of the week and make those your fasting days.

There are a number of researches concerning the 5:2 diet plan, nonetheless thinking of it is a regular fast will absolutely give the majority of the benefits that you are trying to find.

You will certainly have the capability to get it done without needing to stress about making meals the entire day.

Eat-Stop-Eat diet strategy.

The Eat-Stop-Eat diet plan needs you to stop eating for 24 hours, two times a week. This technique was actually first promoted by Brad Pilon and has, in fact, been a preferred technique to do the intermittent fast for a while. It's feasible to follow this fast while still having one meal a day. Most people will have supper one day and after that, will not consume anything till supper the following day. This allows you to never go an entire day without consuming, while still falling in the 24-hour abstaining period.

You can modify this if you like. If it is a whole lot easier for you to go from morning meal to morning meal or lunch to lunch, you can pick those options. During your fast, you are allowed to have coffee, water, and various other non-caloric drinks to keep you hydrated, nevertheless you're not allowed to have any sort of food at all.

Bear in mind that you are simply not eating for a couple of days a week. When it's time to eat usually, you have to eat the same amount of food that you typically do.

If you were not on a fast, have. This will certainly aid you to reduce weight without harming your body.

The greatest issue with this kind of intermittent fast is that fasting for 24 hours is difficult for a number of individuals. You can ease right into it. You might discover that beginning with a much shorter fast, such as the 16-hour quick, can give some good end results. And then after that, you can stop eating for longer amount of times. Going a whole day without eating can be hard, and also the bulk of individuals choose amongst the various other fasting options to see the same outcomes.

Alternative day fasting.

With this option, you will take a fast every other day. There are a couple of options that you can opt for, and also it will certainly depend upon what can help you. A few of these fasts will enable you to have about 500 calories on your fasting days. You will discover that the majority of the lab research studies concerning Intermittent Fasting used some variant of the alternative day fast to help identify all the wellness advantages.

Fasting every other day can be challenging for lots of people. Requiring yourself to fast every other day can be a challenge. Fasting every other day is something that you will most likely have to do. You will likely feel that you are starving several times a week on this fasting strategy.

Warrior Diet

This is another popular alternative that you can choose for intermittent fasting. It consists of eating percentages of raw fruits as well as veggies throughout the day followed by a huge meal during the night. This requires you to fast throughout the day, taking in just enough to keep you happy, and then feasting in the evening within a four-hour eating home window.

The warrior diet plan is among the first diet plans to consist of some kind of fasting. The warrior diet plan likewise includes food options that mimic the Paleo diet regimen plan. You will not just fast during the bulk of the day and also feast at evening, you will also eat a diet regimen plan that has a lot of unrefined foods that can be found in nature.

Spontaneous Meal Skipping

You can try this if you wish to prepare your body for recurring fasting.

When you can eat, you do not intend to spend much time emphasizing about it. With this fast, you do not need to be anxious about adhering to one of the much more structured Periodic fasting approaches. You will just avoid some dishes periodically.

When you are not hungry or when you are just too busy, you can have a meal. It is a substantial misconception that you need to eat something at all hours to avoid hunger.

The body is well adjusted to manage extensive amount of times without consuming.

Missing out on a few meals, specifically if you are not starving or also active, is not harming to your body.

You are practically not eating. Whenever you wind up avoiding a dish or two, or if you are too busy to order a morning meal on the way out the door, just see to it that you eat a healthy and balanced lunch and also supper. If you are out running duties and you are not able to discover someplace to eat, then it is fine to lose out on a meal.

This is not going to cause any harm and will assist you in saving time.

You most likely won't see as good of a result especially when compared to a few of the other choices, but it is much better than nothing and is a lot simpler to work with, possibly. When it works, attempt to skip a meal or two throughout the week or miss out on some meals.

As you can see, there are different alternatives that you can deal with when you are all set to go on the intermittent fast. Some of these will be easier than others, and some might fit your schedule much better. You will have to select which fast is easier for you to adapt to your life.

Essential Principles For Eating On Intermittent Fasting

Consuming on the intermittent fast can be as simple or as complex as you want. Some people will certainly proceed with their healthy consuming in advance while others will include another kind of diet to see faster results.

Due to the fact that it helps to restrict, ketogenic diet regimen can function quite well with this choice. Carbohydrates can lead to reduced hunger and also shed the fat much more rapidly.

When on an intermittent fast, it is not important for you to go on a certain diet strategy to see outcomes.

Intermittent fast

The first point to bear in mind is that you are not permitted to eat undesirable food when you are on this kind of diet regimen. It is exceptional to lower your window of consuming throughout the day to eight hrs or less (or to do one of the various other alternatives for intermittent fasting). If you spend that time consuming meals and fast foods, you will run into problems.

At first, you will not have the capability to decrease weight when you consume by doing this. Quick foods as well as various other unhealthy selections feature great deals of calories per serving, also it's likely that you are absorbing more than one offering at once. Even your window for eating is smaller sized, you can still absorb a whole lot of calories which will stop all your weight-loss progression. Despite the truth that intermittent fasting is not about the calorie-intake, you still have to be mindful about it because it's a component that can impact your eating and calories.

The effectiveness of periodic fasting

You will also find that when you consume these unhealthy foods, even while on an intermittent fast, you will certainly not improve your health. Your health will depend on food high in nutrients to keep you strong. Fasting while still consuming unhealthy food, will likely create various concerns as you discovered prior to starting the fast.

You will certainly notice that you are starving much more frequently when you take in these negative foods and you will fight to endure your fasting durations. This is because great deals of processed and quick foods include preservatives and also chemicals that are developed to make you starve more often. If you prefer to see the outcomes and also make it through your fast without feeling deprived, then it is time to take in foods that are healthier.

Currently, this doesn't mean that you can't consume sugary foods or refined foods on occasions.

The intermittent fast does not have set guidelines for exactly what you are enabled to consume, it just sets the times that you are permitted to consume. Consuming a little rip off dish is fine, as long as you have it during your eating home windows and also just do it now and then. It could be challenging usually but taking in much healthier foods will provide you with far better results. The trick to making the intermittent fast work for you is to eat a healthy diet plan.

The more nutrients you can include into your diet strategy, the much better benefits you will end up getting with this fast.

The first thing that you need to put into consideration is consuming fruits and vegetables as much as possible. Because it supplies lots of vitality, fresh produce is best nutrients that your body needs to stay healthy. Think about filling your plate with vegetables and fruits each meal so that you are getting the nutrients that you require. Eating a wide array of products is likewise essential to ensuring that you are getting what your body requires without including too many calories.

Next, you should go with some excellent sources of protein. You must consider opting for alternatives like lean ground turkey, beef, and chicken. Having some bacon and other fatty meats on occasion is fine, just don't overdo it. Consuming a great deal of fish will give you the healthy fatty acids that the body needs to function correctly.

Healthy and balanced resources of dairy help you to remain lean while providing your body the calcium it requires. You can have some options such as milk, yogurt (be cautious of the kinds that have fruit as well as other things included considering that these usually contain a high amount of sugar), sour lotion, cheese, and so forth. Ensure to check the salts and also sugars that are not healthy and balanced for the body.

You are allowed to have some carbohydrates on this diet. Because due to the fact that lots of diet plans recommend that you avoid them, carbohydrates have actually gotten a little bit of a negative record.

The important thing below is to eat the carbohydrates that are healthy and balanced for you. White bread and pasta are basically sugars in camouflage and need to be avoided.

When it comes to your carbohydrates, using entire grain and whole wheat choices guarantee that you can get all the nourishment that you need.

Having a well-balanced diet will certainly be vital to ensuring that you really feel excellent when you get on an intermittent fast. You will be able to mix up the meals that you select, so you obtain the best results when you take this kind of a fast.

You are also allowed to have a treat, as long as you are cautious with just how often this takes place. If you are eating junk, you will be disappointed when you go to the scale and see that you are not dropping weight. You can have them on occasion, but make sure that it is not something that you frequently take while on this diet plan.

Using the ketogenic diet plan with Intermittent Fasting

Many people choose to use a ketogenic diet regimen strategy while doing an intermittent fast to stay healthy. The ketogenic diet plan is a high fat, modest healthy protein and low carbohydrate diet plan that will certainly assist you to melt fat quickly while lessening your dependence on carbohydrates. There is a great deal to like with this diet regimen plan, and when it is incorporated with the intermittent fasting, you are sure to obtain some fantastic outcomes in no time.

It's possible to use both of these diet plans together. Intermittent fasting is focused on the moments of day when you will certainly eat, while the ketogenic diet focuses on what to eat during those time durations. For those that wish to balance their blood sugar level and dream to lose weight extra effectively, integrating these two diet regimen plan techniques together can be amazing.

With intermittent fasting, you limit the hours that you

can consume. Instead of spreading your meals and also your treats throughout the day, you will limit it to some hours. Various people will choose to just take in between 10 as well as six and fit their macronutrients right into that time duration. Others will certainly take two or three days throughout the week to fast and also fit their nutrients into the week.

The point is that you are restricting the amount of time that you eat, compelling you to think more concerning the foods you take in. You similarly get the advantage of even more weight reduction, when you do recurring fasting.

While you have made it possible to eat, you will certainly need to stick to the macro-nutrients that we talked about above that are approved for the ketogenic diet. You will still stick to high fat, moderate protein, and low carb diet plan even while Intermittent Fasting. You will simply need to be more cautious about the times you eat those macronutrients, but otherwise, you can follow the ketogenic diet plan exactly the same.

If you desire to get a few of the advantages of periodic fasting or you desire to boost your weight-loss, then including this diet with the ketogenic diet regimen can be reliable. You can experiment with the various recurring fasting options to see which one fits into your timetable the best or functions the greatest for you. Obviously, if you find the ketogenic diet plan is reliable or intermittent fasting is too hard, you can stick to the ketogenic diet regimen and also not fast and still see superb outcomes.

It is essential to keep in mind that you do not have to adhere to the ketogenic diet regimen plan if you don't wish to while on an intermittent fast. Lots of people choose other healthy and balanced diet regimen plans instead of picking the ketogenic diet regimen strategy. Many people will choose the ketogenic diet since it is easy to follow and will enable them to shed a lot more fat.

Eating on the intermittent fast does not need to be also challenging. You can select the foods that you desire to eat, although it is very crucial to opt for foods that are whole and fresh and will load you up as well as help with the fat burning process to aid you to see the weight-loss that you are searching for.

CHAPTER NINE
Anti-Aging Effect Of Intermittent Fasting

How Fasting Supports Anti-Oxidant Defenses

As humans age, reactive oxygen varieties (ROS) generally increases as our all-natural antioxidant defenses lower. This inequality becomes better with time, as damage accumulates and also mitochondrial disorder becomes more prevalent.

Normal manufacturing of oxidants in particular cell-types works to control pathways (ROS are associated with some signaling procedures), so discovering the right balance as we age is important. This ideal balance may be critical for maximizing mitochondrial performance and is occasionally referred to as mitohormesis, the concept being we need a "simply appropriate" amount of ROS, with inadequacy leading to substandard performance yet high quantities causing damages. This is particularly essential for cells that depend on generating huge quantities of ATP for their metabolism (including mind, heart, and muscular tissue).

One of the understandings that have actually come from mitohormesis is that we require some quantity of ROS to cause flexible actions that regulate antioxidant defenses as well as make cells and mitochondria more capable of dealing with stress and anxiety as well as contaminants." This protein sustains antioxidant defenses via the following:

Regrowth of oxidized cofactors and healthy proteins (re-growing more of the old "good things").

Nrf2 is not the only device that advertises antioxidant defenses and support. Just like all the five devices that we've broken down, they are interrelated and support each other throughout the complex human system.

Not eating for healthspan & lifespan.

The quantity of time we live is called lifespan. The

length of time that an individual is functional and healthy and balanced-- not just alive-- is called healthspan.

Calorie limitation (including periodic fasting, time-restricted consuming, and also prolonged fasting) is beneficial for impacting both life-span (in researched microorganisms but not yet confirmed in people) as well as the healthspan (in organisms including humans).

It is typical within the aging as well as durability room (at the very least through media depictions) to concentrate on lifespan to the detriment of high quality of life.

On the other hand, the size of time that a person is useful as well as healthy and balanced is associated with better quality of life. Healthspan can be mediated by nutritional interventions, workout is an example, but additionally social communication, area, and also family. A study from Innovations in Aging followed 5,000 Japanese participants for over 20 years and ended

"... social communication is favorably associated to longevity as well as a life of complete satisfaction." Healthspan might be better to stress than life-span alone.

Programmed Aging Vs Damages Buildup

Within the aging community, there is a dispute between the significance of set aging vs. damage build-up. As with most physical arguments, humans are complicated systems that most likely involve a combination of both.

Programmed aging describes the changes in just how our genes are expressed as we age. Some are overexpressed and others are underexpressed.

Damages buildup is identified by cellular as well as mitochondrial damages in time.

Both configured aging and also damage build-up take place at the mobile degree with each intensifying the impacts of the other (i.e., modifications in gene expression speed up damage build-up, while damages accumulation impacts a cell's capacity to have healthy and balanced genetics expression).

Aging Benefits of Intermittent Fasting

This scientific review of the mechanisms included with aging and durability is beneficial past the context of fasting. As you will certainly see in our Fasting Q&A, these mechanisms educate nootropics and also other techniques we can make use of to support healthy aging.

Although we have described lots of advantages that occur when we generate some degree of short-lived "starvation," it's worth noting that there's even more than one method to trigger a few of these reactions (see What to Expect While Fasting). It's likewise crucial to understand that some of the benefits happen throughout the fasting period, yet others take place when we start consuming generally again.

A reoccuring style from the American Academy of Anti-Aging Medicine (A4M) conference that was held mid-December 2018 was the pointer that starvation (i.e., fasting) primes the system for rejuvenation, however it is the refeeding that restores the brand-new cells as well as organelles to boost health. Masochistic semi-starvation because it is "excellent" might be recklessness when cycles of modest fasting treatments will do.

Go back to review What to Expect While Fasting for execution strategies if you feel extra persuaded that not eating benefits are worthwhile to explore. In our Q&A on Fasting we address usual questions as well as help to make fasting as useful and also sustainable and feasible.

CHAPTER TEN
Basic Tips For Intermittent Fasting

Achieving success with Intermittent Fasting can take time. You will need to change a few of the eating patterns that you are used to, but it can be reliable for you in many ways. You will certainly see that it is much easier to slim down, boost your energy, shed body fat, get even more done, and protect against diseases such as diabetic issues, mental deterioration, and cancer cells.

Intermittent fasting is easier than a great deal of other diet regimen strategy prepares out there, it still takes some work. A few of the points to keep in mind to get the most out of your intermittent fast are:

Drink lots of water: Water keeps you hydrated as well as makes you full.

When you get on your fast, you really feel fuller. Remaining in a fasted state functions as a diuretic, which recommends that your body will normally remove water at a much faster price than are utilized to. What all of it comes down to is that you are going to consume a gallon of water a day for the best results.

Consume tea and coffee: When you are really feeling hungry, you may discover that it's useful to drink tea or coffee to lower your food cravings.

Caffeine is a natural suppressant. Just attempt not to take in any caffeine close to bedtime (a minimum of 3 hours), or you may have trouble sleeping.

Keep yourself busy: You might discover that you are extra efficient on an empty tummy. If you are keeping yourself active, you will not just get even more done, you'll also have the capacity to distract yourself from hunger. If you do not find reliable means to fill your time initially, then you will find that the hours you are not eating can seem to expand right into days. Don't make things harder on your own than they need to be.

When it worries the early days of your new consuming technique, ensure your days are full of activities.

Make it flexible: There are numerous selections that include recurring fasting. You do not need to go with one option since everybody else is. You can blend and match as well as develop the routine that benefits you. Periodic fasting is all about having the flexibility to do it the way you desire.

Try it for a minimum of a month: You need a minimum of 3 to 4 weeks to know if the intermittent fast is right for you. If you do not do it for this long, you are not supplying the body the moment it requires to adjust, and you are not offering it an affordable shot. Try it out for at the very least this quantity of time to see if it's the ideal option for you.

Attempt other fasting methods: What helps one person may not help you. If you notice that specific fasting times are better than another version of intermittent fasting and much more reliable, select those. It's all experimenting to see what really feels right for you.

Postpone your morning meal gradually: One thing that works well for a good deal of people is to gradually delay their morning meal. By progressively pushing back your morning meal time an hour weekly or two, you will ultimately get used to an intermittent fast without it being too tough. If you generally eat breakfast at 8 am, wait until 8:30 am to consume your morning meal, for the very first week push your morning meal back to 9 and continue in week 2.

Proceed with this up until your very first meal occurs around twelve noon, take in water in the early morning. Often when you really feel like you are starving in the morning, it is because you have really gone all night without consuming. A terrific behaviour to start is to drink a glass of water right when you awaken in the morning.

Include weights: If you are attempting to slim down and condition, it makes sense to include some weightlifting to your routine. While you will certainly not want to mix things up too much when you first starting, when your body has actually adjusted to the Intermittent fasting way of life, there is no reason you should not take things up a notch.

You will certainly be stunned at what your body can manage if you take things gradually. Ultimately you must have the ability to manage a full intensity.

Enjoy: With recurring fasting, you need to understand that you can live it up on party. You can enjoy as long as you guarantee that all of it cancels in the long run. While the average diet regimen is all about the foods that you aren't enabled to consume, an intermittent fasting lifestyle stand for the truth that you cannot prepare your meals frequently.

This indicates that as long as you get your fasting duration in, there is no reason you can't move your hors about, as long as you don't do so continuously. What's even more, there is no element you can't indulge every so often, as long as one decadent and also delicious treat doesn't become 7 or 8.

Leave your home: There is a good deal of temptation in your residence. For that reason, it is better to leave your residence, so you do not eat every one of that food. Even if you have youngsters around, consider a task you all can do to keep yourselves busy.

Consume extra healthy protein as well as healthy and balanced fat: Eating extra protein with each dish makes it easier to manage your cravings and also establish your muscles. Eating extra healthy and balanced fat will certainly supply you extra power and also make you feel fuller for much longer too.

Many thanks to the dangerous development of the Standard American Diet, a large mass of those in the Western world eat far too much carbs and also not enough protein or healthy fat. To correct this problem, begin considering the macros of the foods you consume. Furthermore, make certain that when you are in a consuming window you load your plate with foods that will make sticking it out to the following window as basic as feasible.

Protect against the negative things: You need to see to it that you are not utilizing it as an excuse to eat processed food regularly. Stick with a healthy diet to make sure that you provide your body with enough nourishment, also if you choose to go on a fast. It is extremely essential to remember that a significant component of intermittent fasting is creating up a calorie shortage by the end of the week to sustain added weight loss. If you fill your body with high-calorie junk food which you get in a consuming window, what you are really doing is sabotaging every one of your effort.

Making healthy options at all time will boost the complete performance of your weight-loss efforts. Obviously, there are numerous points you can do to get the most out of intermittent fasting. This does not suggest you need to prepare for continuous weight reduction, nonetheless, despite exactly how rigid your fasting could be. While you will likely see weight reduction at extreme initially as your body adapts to less calories in its system; this will likely stop and begin throughout your time fasting.

The results are particularly visible after the initial couple of weeks of the change as your body tries to hold on to every little thing it has up until it can figure out what is going on. Once it gets with the program, nonetheless, things should continue as anticipated.

Every diet plan is most likely to have periods of fat burning plateau. That is simply a component of weight-loss that cannot be reduced. As long as you stay consistent,

weight-loss will ultimately resume. The most awful thing you can do is to try and adjust things as long as you get weight-loss back on the right track as that will just make it harder for your body to start losing weight again. Rather, if you continue the course and maintain the plan, you will begin seeing outcomes once more before you understand it.

CHAPTER ELEVEN
Understanding Fasting and Your Metabolism

If you have actually followed any of today's popular diets, you might understand that they are all based upon a certain concept. Their story goes like this: if you lower your calories excessiveness briefly, you will stop losing fat because your body has gone into "hunger mode" and your metabolic rate will slow to a grinding halt. In truth, this saying might be the basis for today's weight loss industry which is factually wrong.

Our metabolism, or metabolic rate, is based on the energetic expenses of keeping the cells in our bodies alive. For instance, let's say we put you in a fancy laboratory and measured the quantity of calories you burned sitting on a sofa for hours in a day. Assuming the number was 2,000 calories. This is regarded as the normal metabolic rate; 2,000 calories would be the quantity of calories you need to consume to match the quantity you burn simply being you.

Now, let's say you walked around that day, possibly 30 minutes of strolling. You may burn an extra 100 calories bringing your daily overall number of calories burned up to 2,100. Your basal metabolic rate is constantly 2,000, and then any extra energy you use up moving your body (like when we do a workout) is contributed to that number.

In this situation, you are liable to burn 2,000 calorie daily no matter what you do. Why are we being told that our metabolism will slow down if we do not eat for an extended period of time?

The response lies with an intriguing metabolic procedure of eating called "the thermic impact of food", and some smart analysis of this rather basic procedure.

The act of consuming can increase your metabolic rate by an extremely little quantity, and this is what is known as "the thermic result of food". This speeds up the metabolic rate as a result of the additional energy your body uses to digest and process the food.

It takes energy to break down, digest, take in, and save the food once you consume it. This "energy expense" has been measured in laboratory settings and is the basis for popular diet plans that promote the metabolic expense of one nutrient over another.

For instance, it takes more calories to absorb protein than to absorb carbs or fats, so some diets recommend replacing some protein for carbs and fat presuming this will burn more calories. This is scientifically true, the quantity of extra calories this dietary change will cause you to burn is really little and will hardly make a difference to your overall calories burned at any given day.

Take for instance, the idea of eating an additional 25 grams of protein so you can burn more calories can appear somewhat outrageous. If you consume an extra 25 grams of protein, you would be including 100 calories to your diet simply so you can burn 10 more calories! The more rational method would be to just not eat those 100 calories.

Nearly all the calories you burn daily result from your resting metabolic rate (the calories it takes just to be alive). Beyond that, the only substantial method to increase the quantity of calories you burn in a day is to exercise and move around.

The research on metabolic rate and calorie consumption is extremely conclusive. I was quickly able to find the following research study that determined metabolic rate in individuals that were either fasting, or on extremely low-calorie diets.

In a research study carried out at the University of Nottingham (Nottingham, England), scientists found that when they made 29 males and females fast for 3 days, their metabolic rate did not change. This is 72 hours without food. So much for needing to eat every 3 hours.

In another study carried out in Pennington Biomedical Research Center, males and females who fasted on a daily basis for 22 days experienced no decline in their resting metabolic rate.

In still more studies, performed on males and females between the ages of 25 and 65, there was no modification in the metabolic rate of individuals who stay away from breakfast, or people who ate two meals a day compared to 7 meals per day.

Eat Stop Eat

In a research study released in 2007, 10 lean men fasted for 72 hours directly. At the end of their fast, their energy expenditure was measured and discovered to be the same from the measurements that were taken at the beginning of the research. Yet another example showing that fasting does not reduce or slow one's metabolic process.

The fact is, food has little to do with your metabolism. Your metabolic process is much more carefully connected to your bodyweight than anything else. And, your metabolic process is practically exclusively connected to your lean body mass or "LBM". This iindicates all the parts of your body that are not body fat.

The more lean mass you have, the greater your metabolism, and vice versa. It does not matter if you are dieting, dieting and exercising or perhaps following a very low-calorie diet plan. As the chart below illustrates, it is your lean body mass that determines your metabolic process.

The only thing that can affect your metabolic process (in both the brief term and long term) is workout or the complete lack of food for 3 days, your metabolic process remains the same.

This is genuinely a testament to the fantastic power and persuasive nature of the marketing found on the internet and in physical fitness as well as nutrition magazines. It is likewise an illustration of the scientific illiteracy of many fitness characters and marketers you might deal with in your daily life. This got me thinking that if short-term changes in food consumption have no effect on metabolic rate, what other misconceptions have I been led to believe as clinical realities?

I took it upon myself to take a look at the science behind a number of today's popular diet plans. I discovered no difference in any of them in their efficiency over the long term.

Individuals picking greater protein, lower carbohydrate diets (comparable to Atkins or The Zone) tended to see slightly much better weight loss, at least in the brief term. However, when these research studies encompassed more than six months and as much as a year, the distinctions tended to even out.

I discovered one thing to be constant with these diets. This common finding which is the success of any diet can be determined by how carefully individuals can follow the rules of the diet plan and for how long they can preserve calorie constraint.

In other words, a diet plan's success can be measured by how well they can enforce, my nutrition "truth" extended calorie limitation is the only proven nutritional method of weight-loss.

If the diet plan permits you to remain on the diet plan for a long period of time, then you have a great opportunity of achieving success in continual weight-loss.

From what we have seen, there is a large number of science that supports using short-term fasting as an excellent way to bring about dietary limitation, and it appears to be a easy and efficient way to lose body fat (which is preferably the goal of ANY weight reduction program). Above that, we have also identified that short-term fasting does not have a negative effect on your metabolism.

Up until now, so good. Fasting does not trigger any unfavorable or damaging effects on our metabolisms, but leaves us with another unanswered question: what type of effect does brief durations of fasting have on our muscles?

CHAPTER TWELVE
Fasting and Exercise

Your muscle cells have the capability to store sugar in a modified kind called glycogen. The intriguing feature of this procedure is that your muscles lack the ability to pass this saved sugar back into the bloodstream. To put it simply, as soon as a muscle has actually saved up some glycogen, it can just be burned by that muscle and cannot be dispatched for use by other parts of your body.

For instance, the glycogen stored in your ideal leg muscles can only be used by your ideal leg muscles. It cannot be donated to your liver, brain, or any other part of your body. This standard guideline goes for all your muscles. This is against how your liver works. Your liver stores glycogen for the purpose of feeding your brain, organs and other muscles as required.

During fasting your body system are counting on fat and sugar that is saved in your liver for strength. Your muscles still have their sugar that they need for exercising. The sugar in your muscles is utilized up quickly during high intensity exercises like weightlifting and sprinting, but even a couple of successive days of fasting and the lack of workout has little effect on muscle glycogen content. By doing so, your muscle glycogen is genuinely booked for the energy requirements of exercise.

Normally, research has found that any effect that brief periods of fasting has on workout performance is small. Research study completed in 1987 discovered that a 3.5 fast day quickly caused very little problems in physical efficiency steps such as isometric strength, anaerobic capacity or aerobic endurance.

In plain English, they found that a 3-day fast had no unfavorable results on how strongly your muscles can contract, your ability to perform short-term high strength exercises, or your capability to work out at moderate strength for a long period of time.

More research published in 2007 found that doing 90 minutes of aerobic activity after an 18-hour fast was not related to any decline in efficiency or metabolic activity. What makes this study a lot more interesting is not only was fasting being compared to the efficiency of individuals who had actually recently consumed, however it was also being compared against the performance of individuals who were supplementing with carbs during their workouts!

This indicates fasting does not adversely affect anaerobic short-burst workout such as lifting weights, nor does it have a negative impact on common "cardio" training.

The only circumstance where I think there might be an unfavorable impact from fasting is during prolonged sports, such as marathons or Ironman-style triathlons, where you are exercising continually for a number of hours at a time. These types of ultra-long competitions usually require the athletes to consume during the real event in order to preserve performance over such prolonged time durations.

In most research study trials examining the effects of fasting on prolonged endurance activities, it was discovered that fasting negatively impacted both general endurance and viewed exertion. Note that these research studies were performed at the end of a 24-hour fast. So it is not suggested to engage in a 3.5-hour biking right at the end of a 24-hour fast, however I'm hoping you already knew that.

Be aware that the "unfavorable effect" that happens from fasting before a long endurance activity just impacts a professional athlete's time up until exhaustion (performance duration). So, the amount of time a professional athlete can exercise while fasted prior to becoming tired is less than the quantity of time it takes for a fed athlete to become exhausted.

Despite the fact that fasting may decrease the quantity of time it takes for an athlete to become tired, fasting really has other positive effects, one of them being weight loss.

Professional athletes carrying out long endurance activities while fasted actually burn more body fat than athletes who are fed (since the fed professional athletes are burning through food energy before they get to the kept energy in their body fat). Depending on your goals, fasting prior to endurance workout may in fact be advantageous (so much for the idea that you definitely need to eat a small meal prior to working out-- this totally depends on your workout objectives). Outside of these performance-based problems, I see no reason you cannot work out while you are fasting. The obvious anecdotal issue would be issues about exercise throughout fasting being able to trigger low blood sugar levels. This has actually been attended to in research study performed on experienced long range runners.

Remarkably, when the blood sugar levels of the runner's first run and second run were compared, they discovered no difference between blood sugar levels during the two 90-minute runs. Not just this, but the fasting run also led to greater rates of fat burning.

It also took nearly 30 minutes of exercise in the fed-state before the runner's insulin levels fell to the same levels that they had before they even started their run when they were in the fasted state. In other words, after 23 hours of non eating, the racer's insulin rates had fallen to the same rates you would have after 30 minutes of running.

From a health viewpoint, that's quite a fantastic running start!

Here is another fascinating advantage of exercise while fasting. There are metabolic pathways that help in maintaining your blood sugar and glycogen levels while you are fasting, and workout has a favorable impact on these routes.

During high-intensity exercise, your muscles produce a bi-product called lactate (in some cases referred to as lactic acid). Lactate has actually been wrongfully accused of triggering the pain in your muscles when you exercise, and something called delayed start muscle pain, the pain you feel days after your exercise. While lactate does not trigger discomfort, it does assist in maintaining your blood glucose and glycogen levels while you fast.

When lactate levels rise in your muscles due to a workout, it can leave the muscle and travel to the liver where through a process called gluconeogenesis (making new glucose), it is related to healing of glycogen shops. Exercise can help in preserving blood glucose levels and glycogen stores while a person is fasting.

In reality, it's not only lactate that helps to keep your blood sugar and glycogen levels while you fast. The very act of burning fat also launches something called glycerol from your body fat stores. The complimentary fats in your fat shops are connected to glycerol while it is stored in your body fat. When the fats are released, so is the glycerol.

Glycerol is an important precursor for gluconeogenesis in the liver. The act of burning fat can also help in preserving blood glucose and liver glycogen stores. And since low strength workout tends to increase the rate of fat release and the quantity of fat burned as a fuel, you might say that both high-intensity and low-intensity exercise actually assist to make your fasts simpler by helping to regulate your blood sugar level levels, and supply foundation to preserve your glycogen levels.

I believe the instruction to eat prior to an exercise or a difficult activity is more of a mental need than it is a physical need. Fasting has little to no effect on many types of exercise, and exercising while fasting may actually make your fast feel much easier by keeping blood glucose levels and glycogen shops.

Nevertheless, fasting is not recommended before long-length endurance events nor during the training of elite athletes, if the training includes multiple workouts every day and where performance is the primary priority over body composition. However for everybody else the combination of fasting and exercise might be a potent method to lose body fat and keep muscle mass.

The other fantastic myth about dieting and fasting is that you will lose your muscle mass while you diet plan. Based upon the readily available research, this is totally wrong.

Maintaining muscle mass seems to be a very essential thing in the diet plan industry right now and for good reason. Muscle makes up a big percentage of your lean body weight, and for this reason, muscle is a big factor in the amount of calories you burn in a day.

While the idea that muscle burns huge number of calories is a bit of a stretch (every pound of muscle on your body burns about five calories daily, not 50 like typically specified), the reality that you can lose or construct muscle makes the metabolic contribution of muscle really crucial. Not only that, you cannot deny the impact that muscle has on your body image. Being lean AND having muscle definition generally makes people feel excellent about themselves.

Thankfully, not only does minimizing your caloric consumption not cause your metabolic process to decrease, it also does not lead to loss of hard-earned muscle.

There is one imperative rule that goes along with this declaration. You need to be associated with some sort of resistance exercise, such as raising weights. Now, you do not have to weight train at the same time you are fasting, however resistance training should be taking place eventually for your muscle mass to be protected in the face of a caloric deficit.

While long-lasting calorie restriction by itself can trigger you to lose muscle mass (such is the case with hospital clients who are on a low-calorie diet and confined to bed rest), the combination of caloric limitation with resistance exercises has been shown to be very reliable at preserving your muscle mass.

A study discovered that when females and males followed a 12-week diet plan including just 800 calories and around 80 grams of protein each day, they were able to preserve their muscle mass as long as they were working out with weights three times each week.

CHAPTER THIRTEEN
The Eat Stop Eat Way of Life

It is essential to keep in mind right away that I do rule this out as a diet program. There are no stages, no point systems, no weighing foods, and most notably no foods that are off-limits.

I won't tell you that sugar is the cause of your weight problem, because it's not, neither is fat. Part of the reason for our obesity problem is that we're looking for the response in the wrong locations.

Obesity is not produced by one specific macronutrient in our diet plan. In truth, it's not the diet plan at all. In my opinion, the primary reason for our weight problems epidemic is abundance. There is too much food available for us to take in. Like I said earlier, every day in the United States, the food market produces enough food to supply every individual with nearly 4,000 calories (practically double what we normally require in a day).

Integrate this with a highly effective and relentless food marketing market and a misguided and backwards health and nutrition market and the issue ends up being clear. Not only do the majority of us consume too much, however many of us have no idea why.

This is the reason Eat Stop Eat is not a diet; it is a way of life based on the nutritional custom of including the combination of short-term, flexible, and periodic fasting in addition to resistance training in your life.

It's a situation where you accept the impression of taking little 24-hour breaks from consuming, and participating in resistance workouts (exercising with weights) a minimum of 2 to 3 times a week. That's it. Once or twice per week and a commitment to an exercise regimen, the Eat Stop Eat way of life is merely taking a 24-hour break from consuming.

All my research studies has led me to the conclusion that this is the single, finest, and most uncomplicated method to lose weight, to keep muscle, and to enjoy all the incredible health advantages associated with fasting. Bear in mind, quick breaks from consuming are nothing brand-new-- almost everyone fast for 8 to 10 hours every night, so I'm merely asking you to broaden this fast. It is also the simplest way to rid you of obsessive-compulsive eating and the requirement to constantly scour publications and the web for the current and greatest diet plan technique.

With Eat Stop Eat, you fight against obsession and regret that drives a lot of today's eating routines, as we get rid of the idea that you have to be continuously eating, or that there is even one true "ideal" way to eat. The reason I don't consider this design of consuming to be a diet is because unlike nearly all popular diets, the Eat Stop Eat way of life is a sustainable plus to the way we eat.

It is the most convenient way to lose fat, feel in shape, and preserve a lean body as it does not require any challenging nutritional preparation. It does not need special shopping journeys, exotic foods, or costly supplements. It merely asks you to avoid consuming for one or two 24-hour periods weekly.

It is the extremely adaptable aspects of Eat Stop Eat that enable individuals to use it effectively to reduce weight, and it's what allows them to keep the weight off for many years afterwards. If you can't fast for 24-hours every time, don't fret. Twenty-four hours was picked through my research study simply because it was a simple time-frame to bear in mind, enabled individuals to consume every day, and appropriated for all different levels of body fat and weight reduction needs. That being said, there is still an advantage to fasting for 16 hours, or 20 hours. The fact is, as long as you are fasting periodically (while still consuming every day) and resistance training while keeping your way of life flexible, you're doing Eat Stop Eat.

With Eat Stop Eat you are burning fat by doing absolutely nothing: not cooking, not consuming, and not stressing about what you will eat when you're eating. In exchange, you invest a little time raising weights (which you must be doing anyway for the health advantages of workout itself) and attempting to be accountable any time you are consuming.

Above all, with Eat Stop Eat style fasting, you never ever go a day without eating!

How to Fast Eat Stop Eat Style.

In order to fast for 24 hours, you can eat as you usually would till 6:00 pm on the first day, and then fast till 6:00 pm the following day. For example, you might begin your fast on Monday at 6:00 pm and finish it on Tuesday by 6:00 pm. People that use Eat Stop Eat call this a dinner-to-dinner fast.

By fasting in this manner, you manage to consume every day; however you likewise manage to take a 24-hour break from eating. More notably, you break the awful practice of continuously being in the fed state, thus resetting your metabolic balance between fed and fasted.

You can also change this to fit your own individual

lifestyle. This is how you employ Eat Stop Eat to work for you. Try my individual favorite time frame and go 2:00 p.m. to 2:00 p.m. (aptly called the lunch-to-lunch fast) if a dinner-to-dinner fast does not work for you. Keep in mind, the Eat Stop Eat lifestyle is developed to be really flexible. The main thing is to make sure you are sleeping during the parts of the fast that you find most difficult. As an example, if you discover the beginning of a fast more difficult than completion, then you might wish to attempt fasting from 8 p.m. to 8 p.m. It is this versatility that makes Eat Stop Eat so simple. If you were preparing on starting your fast on Tuesday but something happened and you had to go to supper with friends on Tuesday night, there is no need to fret because you can just begin the fast the next day.

Likewise, bear in mind that as your life changes so must your fasts. A dinner-to-dinner fast may be perfect for you when you initially begin fasting, but after a couple months you might find yourself having a difficult time completing your fasts, or feeling a strong desire to eat way too much after you fast. The quickest and easiest option is to try a different fast time. This minor modification can have dramatic outcomes on keeping your fasts both easy and reliable. Constantly test brand-new fast times prior to attempting longer fasts. Keep in mind, keeping it flexible is crucial to long-term sustained weight-loss.

Another crucial aspect of Eat Stop Eat design fasts is that you do drink during your fasts. Throughout your fasts you may consume any calorie-free beverages you like.

As an example, these are all beverages that would be acceptable throughout your fast:

- Black Coffee

- Black tea

- Green tea

- Natural tea

- Water

- Carbonated water

If you are the type that consumes diet soda), even diet plan soda pop. Remember that a significant portion of your daily liquid intake originates from the water in the food you consume, and since you're not consuming when your fasting, it is advisable to drink a little bit more than you typically would.

Attempt your best to keep your calories as near to zero as possible. Once you start including a "bit" of cream and sugar to your coffee, or a "little sip" here or there you may discover that your calorie intake slowly begins to increase throughout your fast. Do your best to get a "no tolerance method" during your fast.

When it pertains to what else you can eat throughout your fasts, follow this standard-- the true advantage is taking breaks from eating, not to determine how to " game the system".

I frequently get concerns about consuming a "bit" of beef broth, or coconut water, or xylitol, or other practically calorie-free foods when having a fast. There is no research to answer questions on the metabolic result of a percentage of calories from all the various food and active ingredient sources. So, remember that calorie-free beverages are alright throughout your fasts, and calorie-free gum is all right in small amounts, however try to avoid any other practically calorie-free foods. The secret is to take a break from eating, not to continue to enhance the pattern of constantly eating and always being fed.

Pertaining to what you can and can't consume during fasting, employ the following guidelines:

If you can go without then go without, however if you really can't go without then do not.

If you are ill, or aren't feeling well, then you do not have to fast. If work gets hectic or you've increased your exercise volume a lot that fasting isn't practical for an amount of time, do not fast. Eat Stop Eat is a versatile long-term solution. On some weeks you might fast once, others two times. It's all about you and your individual preferences. Just do what works for you!

To start, attempt one fast weekly. Experiment with times that work for you best. Once you have the hang of fasting, you can increase the quantity of times each week that you fast. Prevent the errors of attempting to fit as many fasts in a week as possible, or extending your fasts far beyond 24 hours. As I mentioned earlier, I have actually discovered that 24-hours one or two times a week is the flexible and practical way to quickly burn fat.

Extending beyond this greatly lowers the flexibility of Eat Stop Eat and may cause a sort of "fasting burnout". Forcing yourself to fast frequently or for too long to the point where you are dreading your next fast totally beats the purpose of the Eat Stop Eat way of life.

The same goes for fasting more frequently, as I'll be discussing, the benefits of fasting don't just come from the time you are fasting, but likewise the time after the fast. Similar to exercise, there need to be healing time for you to get the full impact. That's why I advise a minimum of 48-hours of time between each 24-hour fast.

After talking with literally thousands of people who have actually been following Eat Stop Eat, I have actually seen that the individuals who remain flexible and relaxed see the best weight loss outcomes and are the most able to keep the weight off. On the other hand, the individuals who try to accelerate the process by fasting several times weekly or extending their fasts to 48 or perhaps 72-hours do see quick results, but they also "stress out" really rapidly.

This is in agreement with the research study on restrained eating, which eloquently reveals that the more restrained an individual is with their consuming, suggesting the more rules they try and follow (excellent food/bad food lists, food combining, etc.), the most likely they will see quick weight-loss, and also the more likely they will experience severe weight rebounds after they have broken some of their rules and restraints. Under comparable conditions, the more restrained you are with your fasts, the more likely you will feel guilty if you break your guidelines and end up overindulging.

The fact is, the Eat Stop Eat way of life must free you from obsessive-compulsive consuming, but this ought to not be at the expense of obsessing about your fasting.

The same "fasting burnout" occurs to individuals who integrate fasting with rigorous dieting, or extreme amount of exercise. As a rule of thumb, if you experience difficulties in organizing fasting, working out, and dieting into your schedule you are more than likely doing too much of one of these activities.

I 'd like you to perform weightlifting at least two times each week, and you can add in cardio-style training if you want, just ensure you are adequately recuperating from your exercises and fasts. With concerns to dieting, as a general rule, if you are fasting, then on the days you are consuming you should not be in any more than a 10% to 20% deficit for any length of time. Your once-

or-twice-per-week fasts are implied to be a replacement for conventional dieting. If you have a significant quantity of weight to lose then you might have the ability to handle both fasting and consuming at a minor deficit, however the leaner you get, the less this is advised. Remember, the goal is not 0% body fat.

Consider fasting as the simplest way possible to get outcomes. Essentially you are getting a rise from not doing anything, so you do not need to make it any more complex than a periodic break from eating, but you ought to go out of your method to view each and every single complete fast as a "mini-victory"-- favorable reinforcement at its best.

CHAPTER FOURTEEN
Why Not Longer Fasts?

There are reasons I prefer 24-hour fasts over longer fasts. One is the ease and simplicity of 24-hour fasts; another is that they enable individuals to still consume every day. I also believe the objective needs to be to balance the times spent fed and fasted, instead of to totally get rid of eating for days on end.

To understand the main reason I do not promote the idea of longer fasts I'm going to need to introduce you to the reciprocal relationship that exists in your body between your weight loss metabolism and your carbohydrate burning metabolism.

In order to satisfy the energy requirements of an average day, your body will burn a mix of fats and carbohydrates. In the resting state (not working out), this mix will largely be figured out by the mix of carbohydrates and fats in your diet. As you slowly begin to go into the fasted state, this blend will gradually favour fat over carbs, and this is for good reason.

As I pointed out previously, when you fast for brief periods of time, your blood sugar level remains stable. It will drop from the high levels that you generally have after consuming a meal, down to what we call fasted levels and after that stay there. We have actually understood this since 1855, when scientist Claude Bernard discovered that throughout the preliminary phases of fasting, the blood sugar level was kept regular due to the breakdown of the liver glycogen.

Liver glycogen (the sugar being stored in your liver) is what keeps your blood sugar level stable at normal levels while you are fasting for brief time periods. If you keep fasting eventually your liver glycogen will begin to run out, and other compensatory systems must come in to play to maintain your blood sugar levels.

As you fast, you gradually get in a fasted state metabolic process-- a metabolism based around activating and utilizing your body fat as a fuel. Fasted state metabolism is a fat-burning metabolic process-- utilizing fat (and later on ketones) as fuel in order to maintain your blood glucose levels and your body protein shops. This is true throughout brief 12 to 24-hour fasts and much longer fasts.

The longer you fast, the greater the modifications that should be made to guarantee that you are able to burn as much fat as possible. In other words, the longer your fast, the more fat loss controls carb burning. Once you are this far into fat loss, you merely cannot turn it off like a switch when you start consuming once again. And this is where a few of the scare about longer term fasting originates from.

Particularly, a boost in blood complimentary fatty acid levels is well known to press your muscles towards oxidizing a high amount of fat as a fuel, but in doing so it must also inhibit glucose oxidation. This change starts very early during a fast, as early as the 8 to 10-hour mark, and then gradually progresses as the level of totally free fats develop in your blood and the level of glycogen reduces in your liver.

There is no genuine way around this. You can't have your muscles likewise burn high quantities of carbohydrates if you desire your muscles to burn your body fat as a fuel. And since your muscles are not oxidizing carbohydrates, less glucose is really entering your muscles. It's still in your blood, but your muscles do not desire any. They are "full" from a carbohydrate viewpoint-- there would be no location to put the glucose if it entered your muscles.

As a result, it is a well-established fact that longer periods of fasting (48 to 72-hours and beyond) do not just induce a high level of fat oxidation, but also produce a short period of insulin resistance at the muscular level in the immediate hours after the quick is finished.

Now, this does not take place throughout a 24-hour fast as it takes around 24-hours just to deplete liver glycogen levels, once glycogen has actually been depleted and the levels of fat in your blood are increased, modifications begin to strike to ensure that your blood sugar levels still remain steady, even in the face of decreased glycogen shops. This appears to take place earlier in ladies than in males, potentially due to the truth that ladies have higher levels of fat in their blood and a much better ability to burn fat while in the fasted state. Basically, ladies go into fasted state metabolic process quicker than males.

When you fast for prolonged periods (two to three days and beyond) your body goes into a kind of permanent fat burning physiology which includes a down regulation of the hormones and enzymes responsible for carb burning.

Usually, this isn't a concern since throughout brief fasts we start to get in the fasted state and increase the amount of fat we burn, however we start consuming again before the body can make up for these preserved elevations in weight loss by decreasing insulin level of sensitivity.

When you considerably pass 24-hours of fasting by 2 to 3-fold, this reduced level of sensitivity to insulin can increase and carry over to when you are consuming. Towards completion of longer-term fasts, your body will launch far more fat into your bloodstream than you can actually use without including some form of workout. So, although you've ended your fast and ate, it's not as if all of those FFA that were released from your body fat shops unexpectedly vanish-- they require a long time to either be burned as a fuel, or restored as body fat.

Now, if for some reason all of these modifications were to immediately reverse after your first bite of a meal after your fast, you would experience some very nasty repercussions. You'd run the risk of becoming hypoglycemic; you'd likewise have a very high fat level in your blood with no method to get rid of that fat, except to re-shop it all immediately as body fat. Neither one of these are ideal situations and for these reasons it takes your body a time period (numerous hours) to come back into a regular state with typical levels of insulin sensitivity after longer fasts.

Fasting for 72-hours can momentarily blunt insulin's ability to prevent lipolysis even in the fed state. This highlights the transition state that happens after a longer fast. The raised levels of development hormonal agent that are released into your blood following a longer-term fast does not vanish the minute you take a bite of your very first meal, and can in fact take numerous hours to reverse to non-fasting levels.

So as you "ramp up" into fat burning mode in a fast, you likewise need to "ramp down" at the end of a fast. However, it's also been found that after this intense period of insulin resistance your body may in fact go back to a level of improved insulin sensitivity, as durations of longer fasting are related to improvements in insulin level of sensitivity when determined a number of days later.

The fact is, there is a significant switch from glucose oxidation to fat oxidation that takes place throughout fasting, and this switch needs some time to emerge. What may not be noticeable is that this switch needs a similar period of time to be undone when re-feeding commences. To put it simply, there is a gradual transition into fasted state metabolic process and there is a steady transition back into fed state metabolic process. The longer the time invested in the fasted state, the longer it takes to return to the fed state.

In the end, I'm unsure how short periods of severe insulin resistance affect human health, some people have even argued that they are good for long-term health and anti-aging.

These are just a few of the reasons Eat Stop Eat is based around short 24-hour durations of fasting. There is ease and flexibility connected with 24-hours of fasting divided between two days, however this ease and versatility is removed when you begin to fast for longer amount of times.

The bottom line is that nearly everyone can fast for 24-hours, but not everybody can do more. For that factor,

24-hours once or twice weekly, separated by 2 to 6-days of regular, accountable eating and routine workout is the Eat Stop Eat prescription for weight loss and total health.

CHAPTER FIFTEEN
Designing Your Own Workout Program

In many research trials where people on a low-calorie diet preserved lean mass by utilizing resistance training, their exercises suit the following parameters: they generally worked out 3 to 4 times each week with each exercise session lasting about 45 minutes. On average, 2 to 3 muscle groups would be exercised per exercise session. Each workout included between 6 to 10 workouts with each exercise being completed for 2 to 4 sets of 8 to 12 reps. Rest durations would consist of approximately 2 minutes rest between each set of a workout.

As I discussed earlier, it is necessary to pick the exercise style that fits your own specific objectives and needs. This is the primary reason that I cannot prescribe an exercise for everyone who follows the Eat Stop Eat way of life.

For example, it takes a high number of weight, volume, and tension for a 250-pound bodybuilder to keep a high rate of muscle mass. If a 250-pound weightlifter were to comply with Eat Stop Eat, the amount and type of workout that he would require to do to preserve his muscle mass would be much higher than what a 145-pound woman who hasn't formerly exercised would need to do. Even more, a 145-pound woman who hasn't formerly worked out in this manner would see extremely little advantage from immediately following the bodybuilder's workout routine.

Selecting the proper exercise program depends on the list below:

- Your current training status (just how much you currently work out).

- Your goals (preserve or get muscle).

- The amount of muscle mass you presently have.

An easy general rule would be to look at the quantity of workout you were doing before following Eat Stop

Eat, and make certain to slowly progress from there. Much like your nutrition program, your exercise regimen ought to focus on the simplest approaches that get you the results you desire.

The Importance of Sticking with It.

If you are relatively non-active, then starting a workout program may in fact be extremely tough. Research has recommended that as many as 50% of people who begin a brand-new workout program will leave within six months. Most times, individuals state the reason that they stop working out is that they are worn out or because of lack of time. It is very crucial that you stick with your program.

Not only will adhering to your exercise program assist you in maintaining muscle mass while you are losing body fat, however, it will also keep your state of mind elevated. In some very intriguing research study published in 2008, it was found that when a group of females who exercised regularly were forced to stop exercising for 72 hours, there was a visible decline in their body satisfaction and state of mind. The outcome of this study also revealed that after 72 hours of non-exercise, feelings of sluggishness, stress, and anxiety were increased. Of course, this is paradoxical since these are the specific reasons most individuals stop working out in the first place.

When you give up an exercise routine, this leads to the concept of a downward spiral. You stopped due to the fact that you were worn out or stressed out, only to become even more exhausted and a lot more stressed, and then the spiral increases in momentum, and you end up glued to your couch without considering the tension of restarting another workout program.

Concerning exercise, balance seems to be the secret. Too much workout and you increase the risk of overuse injuries and you could become compulsive, defining yourself as an individual by your exercise program. Too little workout and you lose the muscle keeping and myriad of health benefits. Not only this, but you likewise risk ending up being disappointed with your body, in addition to experiencing a reduced mood.

For Eat Stop Eat the goal is to utilize workout as a tool. Doing the amount needed to develop some muscle or maintain, but not becoming obsessive to the point where workout disrupts your life. You must look forward to your next exercise session, not fear it. And never ever let it define who you are as a person.

For this reason, I suggest keeping your exercise plans as straightforward as possible. Promote your muscle following the idea in the above paragraphs, permit them to recuperate, then repeat when you are all set.

CHAPTER SIXTEEN
Cardio Training for Weight Loss.

The objective of the Eat Stop Eat way of life is to let the combination of a sensible diet and brief periods of fasting lead to a reduction in body fat, while using resistance training to increase the size or preserve of your lean body mass. While conventional cardio training will not sabotage your weight loss gotten from following Eat Stop Eat, you may be shocked to see that it does not typically produce as big of a weight loss advantage as you may have been led to think. This doesn't imply that cardio is bad for you or a wild-goose chase. Cardio training may be of advantage to your health, it may not pack as much fat burning punch as some people want it.

Presently the suggestion for grownups is to take part in a minimum of 150 minutes of moderate-intense physical activity weekly. This seems like a reasonable suggestion. Nevertheless, I have actually discovered from both individual experience and from evaluating scientific research study that the work-to-reward benefit of cardio for the function of burning more fat is relatively low. This does not mean that cardio doesn't work. Rather, it implies you have to do a disproportionately large quantity of work in the fitness center to get obvious fat-burning results. To put it simply, it might help with fat burning, however you better be prepared to invest a big amount time to get this benefit.

Believe it or not, most research trials analyzing the weight loss triggered by very low-calorie diet plans found that adding workout did little to increase weight reduction beyond what the diet plan alone might attain. To put it simply, when it came to the real weight reduction advantages-- the diet plans appeared to do all the work.

Take, for instance, the research carried out by Donnelly et al. published in 1991. Sixty-nine overweight women were placed on a severe 520-calorie-per-day diet plan (this is much lower than I would ever advise). The ladies were then divided into four groups:

- Group 1 did not exercise.

- Group 2 did endurance workout for 60 minutes, 4 days each week.

- Group 3 did strength training, 4 days weekly.

- Group 4 Strength training and mobility workouts is conducted 4 days a week.

At the end of the 90-day research trial all four groups lost a large quantity of bodyweight, averaging over 40 pounds of weight reduction! The intriguing finding was that there were no differences between the four groups in regards to the body fat that was lost. This is in spite of the massive quantities of working out that the women in Group 4 were doing compared to Group 1!

This conclusion has been discovered over and over again in published research study. Donnelly and co-workers did a second trial, published in 1993 showing that weightlifting might increase muscle size while ladies followed an 800-calorie-per-day diet, however, it might not enhance weight-loss or fat loss. Similar outcomes have actually been discovered by research performed by Janssen in 2002, Kraemer in 1997, Bryner in 1999, and Wang in 2008, just among other examples.

Exercising for weight loss has been studied thoroughly and repeatedly proven to be less effective than we think.

Uncovering the reason exercising for weight reduction performs so poorly in scientific trials have proven to be very difficult. We understand that extra workout does develop a bigger calorie deficit (because workout burns calories). This additional deficit does not seem to show up on the weight loss side of the journal, therefore either the deficit isn't as large as we thought, or there is payment happening somewhere else in our lives.

We also understand that individuals who regularly perform cardio or endurance design training end up being able to burn a higher amount of fat as fuel by regulating enzymes responsible for moving fat into their muscles, and enzymes responsible for burning once it gets in the muscle. In a series of human experiments, it was found over and over that while non-trained muscle only slightly increase their capability to uptake fatty acids to be utilized as a fuel throughout workout, an endurance trained muscle can constantly increase their uptake of fats to a much higher degree. This adjustment seems to occur really rapidly, ending up being substantial after only 8 weeks of endurance training. Yet, we still do not see the extra fat loss we would expect from including cardio to a weight-loss program.

The most apparent response is that exercise just causes people to eat more later in the day. The saying "work up an excellent appetite" appears to support this idea. Medical research study suggests that this is not the case.

An evaluation published in 2003 suggests that women and men can tolerate exercise-induced severe power deficits and do not compensate by eating more later on in the day. Other studies have actually found that this applies for both lean 280 and obese 281 individuals.

Another line of research even suggests that workout might even assist control prompts to binge and eat in reaction to unfavorable emotions, and overall, seem to have a much better control of their appetite.

So while it may hold true for some people, research suggests that for many individuals, workout does not trigger you to consume more calories. The other tip is that workout can develop a decreased quantity of motion in the period after the workout. In research, we call this "spontaneous exercise".

To offer you a very unrefined concept of the theory it would look something like this: on the days that you exercised you likewise invested slightly more time resting on the couch, possibly climbed up the stairs of your house a couple times less, and then took less total actions. These little reductions in spontaneous physical activity may decrease a few of the benefit of the workout. This has actually likewise proven to be really difficult to measure in a research setting.

The real response is most likely a mix of all of these theories. The calorie burn from exercise is merely less than we expect (or wish to believe) and small changes in post-exercise spontaneous physical activity and increase in calorie intake all play a part in making workout less reliable than we would like.

Despite the misleading cause, the reality remains that exercise seems to be less efficient than we want to think. Nevertheless, as I stated in the past, this does not mean workout is useless for weight loss.

A single bout of exercise promotes fat blood circulation and fat mobilization, culminating in the supply of fatty acids to the skeletal muscles at a rate that is compliant with metabolic requirements. During workout (training), there are changes in adipose tissue physiology, especially an improved fat mobilization throughout intense exercise. Epidemiological observations support the concept that physically active people have fairly low fat mass.

Workout likewise appears to be able to cause preferential weight reduction in the visceral fat deposits, more so than either resistance exercise or just calorie constraint. So for people who keep a large amount of fat viscerally, workout may be an important addition to their weight loss program. Maybe workout is not triggering more weight loss, however, but a slightly better circulation of fat loss.

The mistake to cardio training is that similar to weight, fasting, and dieting training, it is a type of stress being put on the body, and too much tension can have deleterious effects. Undoubtedly, persistent exhausting exercise has actually been linked to hypercortisolism, hypogonadism, and nutritional exhaustion. So while the correct amount of cardio can cause significant increases in insulin sensitivity and the increased capability to clear fat from your blood stream to be utilized as a fuel, excessive workout can cause negative health issues, particularly when coupled with a big calorie deficit.

The truth is if you get your diet correctly and are following a nutrition program that allows you to reduce your caloric consumption, it will cause you to drop weight. Including calorie burning exercises does not seem to increase this weight loss to as big a degree as we would like, but might cause small improvements in both weight reduction and health. Including strength training is still the top concern for anybody trying to lose body fat given that it can maintain or even help in increasing the size of your muscles while you are dieting, and prevent undesirable changes in your metabolic process.

For those people who have time or particular requirement, including additional cardio can still be an added fat loss advantage, if you have the time.

The bottom line when it comes to Eat Stop Eat and the Eat Stop Eat lifestyle is the following:

The simple technique is the one that works best, and

this method includes eating for fat loss and exercising to preserve (or even boost) the size of your muscles. Attempt to be as active as possible, while also permitting yourself adequate recovery time. Include cardio just as needed, only if you discover it enjoyable, and have the offered time.

CHAPTER SEVENTEEN
Fasting and Women (Special Considerations)

It must not come as a surprise that there are obvious gender differences in how the body works. From the way they look to their own unique metabolisms, women and men do have varied physiologies.

In brief, aside from the differences in muscle mass and body fat levels, males and females also differ due to ladies having their own set of unique metabolic and physiologic requirements that relate to their child-bearing physiology, and this reality just cannot be overlooked when going over diet plan and weight loss.

In basic, when comparing males and females, women tend to burn more fat on a daily basis and be more insulin delicate than men. Ladies also have very different hormone profiles. There are the obvious differences in sex hormonal agents like testosterone and estrogen which impact not only our capability to burn fat and build muscle, but also affect where we save our body fat.

There are likewise large differences in some of the more vital weight loss hormonal agents. Males tend to have less flowing development hormonal agent than females, and women tend to have 2 to 3-times more leptin than males. A guy's hormone levels also tend to be more steady than a lady's given that many hormones tend to vary within a female's menstruation.

The reality that both leptin and growth hormonal agent are greater in ladies may involve the higher estrogen levels discovered in ladies' bodies. It has been revealed in healthy post-menopausal and pre-menopausal females that estrogen increases blood GH levels. In reality, the combination of high estrogen and high growth hormone is among the hallmark hormonal markers of healthy girls. A healthy girl might secrete anywhere from 2 to 7-fold more GH than pre-pubertal ladies, males, or post-menopausal women.

Due to the fact that of these hormone distinctions women will have higher quantities of totally free fatty acids in their blood compared to a guy after longer periods of fasting (40 to 72-hours). These raised levels of free fats will trigger a female to stay in an increased state of weight loss longer than a man for the duration, after the fast has actually been broken. This appears by the increased fat oxidation even after a meal, slower glucose clearance, and the decreased capability for raised insulin to push a lady out of fat loss during the hours following a fast.

It is real that ladies have a physiology that is uniquely their own, and many of these distinctions include some of the most essential fat-burning hormonal agents. How does this affect their capability to diet plan and lose unwanted body fat?

It is popular that prolonged food deprivation, big energy deficits created through vigorous exercise, and quick weight-loss all might lead to numerous forms of menstrual dysfunction in some (but not all) females.

This is typically seen in women who are dieting for extended periods of time in addition to female professional athletes who are not actively dieting, but not able to satisfy the caloric requirements of their rigorous athletic program.

However, it's not simply prolonged time periods in large calorie deficits that are the problem but having insufficient fat might be an issue for some females in and of itself. In 1974, Frisch and McArthur theorized that the upkeep of normal menstrual function was connected to an important level of 22% body fat. And while the "healthy" quantity of body fat is most likely a range than it is a hard, quick number like 22%; the truth stays, and bears repeating, that the objective of any diet plan program is not to obtain 0% body fat (I know this is apparent, however it needs to be mentioned loudly and typically). Or put in a different way, no matter whether you are a lady or a guy, young or old, bad things start to happen when your body fat levels end up being too low.

For men, the critical level of body fat appears to be closer to 4-6%, but this also seems to vary somewhat based upon age and ethnic background. Both guys and ladies have healthy levels of body fat under which metabolic/hormonal issues may develop, with the levels for guys being less than half that of women.

Research on elite national level woman professional athletes has actually shown that the mix of low body fat levels with a big calorie deficit can result in amenorrhea (absence of their monthly period), in addition to decreased leptin and estradiol levels.

In this study, 39 nationwide level female professional athletes were taken a look at. The leanest ladies tended to be the ones who were amenorrhoeic, and had the most affordable levels of leptin, estradiol, and insulin. These females were roughly 23 years of ages, had a BMI of approximately 18 with a body fat level of around 15%. As an example, a 5' 6" lady in this research study would weigh around 112 pounds, burn nearly 1,000 calories daily through exercise, while eating around 1,700 calories per day and just 55 grams of protein every day.

The females who still had typical menstruations had somewhat more body fat (15.5%), the very same quantity of lean mass, however consumed almost 500 more calories a day, and considerably more protein (78 versus 55 grams daily). They also had higher levels of leptin, insulin, thyroid hormones, and leptin than their amenorrhoeic counterparts.

Although these ladies were not fasting, this study shows that minimal levels of body fat, integrated with long-lasting calorie deficits, and possible moderate protein malnutrition can lead to marked hormonal disruptions.

CHAPTER EIGHTEEN
Meal Plan Guide

Creating a right dish technique you can comply with on your fasting days can be challenging with an intermittent fast. Right here are some superb meal strategies you can follow to help make the intermittent fast job a lot better for you.

F a s t D a y P l a n 1

Breakfast: Quaker Oats sachet of gruel (40g) - 255 calories

Dinner: Beetroot and feta salad - 125 calories

Beetroot (50g) - 13 calories

Feta (30g) - 83 calories

Spinach (60g) - 29 calories

A slice of lemon - 0 calories

Snack: Sliced apple with 1 tablespoon of almond butter - 145

Overall calorie count: 525

F a s t D a y Pl a n 2

Morning meal: Sweet plums with yogurt - 145 calories

100g low-fat all-natural yogurt - 65 calories

2 plums - 60 calories

1 tsp of honey - 20 calories

Dinner: Ryvita and tuna pieces - 253 calories

2 x preliminary Ryvita cracker breads - 70 calories

Tuna mayo (60g) - 171 calories

Rocket (70g) splashed on the top - 12 calories

Fractured black pepper - 0 calories

Treat: Miso soup - 32 calories

Overall calorie count: 430

F a s t D a y P l a n 3

Morning meal: Soft boiled egg and asparagus - 90 calories

1 egg - 70 calories

5 pieces of asparagus - 20 calories

Salt and pepper to season

Supper: Turkey hamburgers with corn-on-the-cob - 328 calories

Minced turkey with poached little egg, spring onion, garlic and chilli (111g) - 172 calories

1 x corn-on-the-cob - 156 calories

Deal with: A couple of frozen grapes - 60 calories

General calorie matter: 478 calories

F a s t D a y P l a n 4

Breakfast: Packet of Belva Breakfast Biscuits (muesli) - 228 calories

Supper: Roasted veggies with balsamic polish - 261 calories

1/2 courgette, 1/2 aubergine, 1/2 butternut squash, 1/2 red pepper - 247

1 tablespoon balsamic vinegar - 14 calories

A press of lemon - 0 calories

Treat: Harley's sugar-free jelly pot - 4 calories

Overall calorie count: 493

F a s t D a y P l a n 5

Morning meal: spinach omelette - 160

2 x eggs - 140

Spinach leaves (60g) - 20

Salt and pepper - no calories

Dinner: Hummus and also crudities - 175 calories

Hummus (40g) - 123 calories

A vegetable bowl packed with carrots, cucumber, raw pepper - 52 calories

Snack: Edamame beans (60g) with rock salt - 84 calories

Overall calorie count: 419

F a s t D a y P l a n 6

Breakfast: Banana and low-fat yogurt - 177 calories

100g low-fat all-natural yogurt - 65 calories

1 x banana - 112 calories

A sprinkle of cinnamon - no calories

Supper: Turkey busts with bent spinach - 216 calories

1 x turkey breast steak (125g) - 175 calories

1 cup of spinach, prepared and seasoned with salt - 41 calories

Treat: 10g of snacks - 59 calories

Total calorie count: 452

F a s t D a y P l a n 7

Morning meal: Apple, carrot, and ginger shake - 107 calories

1 apple - 55 calories

1 carrot - 52

Raw ginger - no calories

Dinner: Pitta pizza - 178 calories

Weight Watchers wholemeal pitta - 106 calories

25g Extra Light Philadelphia cheese - 40 calories

1 tomato - 32 calories

Combined natural herbs - no calories

Salt and pepper - no calories

Treat: 100g blueberries and a handful of almonds - 137 calories

Total calorie count: 422

CHAPTER NINETEEN
Guide on Eat Stop Eat

By now I hope it clear to you that occasional short periods of intermittent fasting combined with a routine resistance-training program is an easy, straightforward, and highly reliable method to reduce weight. It can likewise help in correcting some of the negative metabolic results that come from spending a lot of time in the fed state, and can enhance many markers of long-lasting health.

To get the full advantage of Eat Stop Eat, remember to include resistance training as part of your weight loss program and overall technique to health. Just how much and what style depends on you, simply keep in mind to always stabilize the quantity of exercise you do with just how much time you need to recuperate from that exercise.

You might also carry out cardio-type exercise with Eat Stop Eat, simply bear in mind that while there are health benefits to this kind of workout, too much can lead to an unfavorable influence on your health.

Never hesitate to adjust the quantity you exercise or how often you fast in order to maintain your energy levels and total feelings of health. Some weeks you might fast two times, others only when necessary. Some weeks you might lift weights four times, others you may just lift only two times. The secret to keeping this lifestyle sustainable is to always remember to keep it versatile and adjust to stresses and needs of your everyday life.

Keep in mind that there is no need to stack Eat Stop Eat on top of other, more stricter kinds of dieting. While many diets tout day-by-day diet plans, cookbooks, and charts of appropriate and unacceptable foods, none of this is needed when you adopt the Eat Stop Eat way of life.

Eat Stop Eat will ideally release you from the nutrition info-clutter that surrounds us every day in the media.

Worrying over what we consume, how we workout, what to do to reduce weight, and all the confusion and frustration that goes along with these things no longer needs to be a part of your life. You do not need any of them to drop weight. Any message that has lots of nutrition and fitness rhetoric and "consume this, not that" lists and rules that "you absolutely need to follow" is nothing more than dietary mind-clutter.

Getting rid of this stress can, in fact, improve your weight loss and overall health. As unexpected as it sounds, "worrying" over your diet can actually make slimming down harder. It has been suggested that excessive mental tension integrated with overeating can really have synergistic results that are harmful to both your weight reduction goals and long-term health.

What is fascinating is that the tension of excessive dietary restraint, particularly when not accompanied by the act of really consuming less can increase markers of stress response within the body. So when I say that "stressing" about eating healthy isn't helpful for you, I mean it in the most actual sense!

In truth, the reproductive hormonal agents in both men (testosterone) and ladies (estrogen) are both highly responsive to not only physical stress, but mental stress as well. So you genuinely can worry yourself into jeopardized health. Now there is an advantage to eat healthy. I'm not offering you a reason to eat like a child the day after Halloween. I still suggest consuming a range of veggies and fruits combined with some sources of protein, but I highlight that in the Eat Stop Eat manner, you do not have to stress over what you choose to eat.

I desire you to eat in a method that is sustainable, and then to take a periodic break from eating in the form of a short fast. It might be one fast per week, or it might be two depending on how you are feeling.

Think of fasting as a passive technique to weight reduction enabling weight loss to happen at its own speed, rather than obsessive amounts of dieting and exercise which aggressively causes your body to lose increasingly more fat, at rate that is always near the upper-limit of what your body can manage.

With fasting, we slim down through the actions of not doing anything, or more particularly through the actions of consuming absolutely nothing. We lose weight when we are not eating. And when we consume, we enjoy eating. The Eat Stop Eat lifestyle can be best described by a little modification of a popular Zen quote:

By following the Eat Stop Eat way of life, you are able to slim down by utilizing a worry-free and uncomplicated style of consuming that balances your fed and fasted metabolic process. This enables you to reap the health and metabolic advantages of brief durations of fasting, consisting of weight loss, reduced inflammation, and enhanced metabolic profile, while lowering the quantity of time you spend thinking about what you are eating.

The fact is that, with Eat Stop Eat, we can slim down while developing a much healthier interaction with food and agree the food is:

When you need it,

a) A fuel for your body, and

b) To be enjoyed.

From this point forward, you can take pleasure in the foods you consume, and delight in understanding that with the Eat Stop Eat way of life you can lose fat, develop muscle, eat every day, never ever follow some crazy fad diet plan ever again, and be 100% favorable that not only is taking the periodic break from consuming okay for you, but that it really has tremendous health advantages.

Consume less, stress less; move more, lift more, and get a great night's sleep. For physical health, that's basically as excellent as it gets.

CONCLUSION

Intermittent Fasting is an exceptional selection if you prefer to shed fat, lower weight, and also have a better shape. This diet plan is not just about the foods that you take in. It is also about the time of the day that you eat these foods to ensure that you can be healthy and balanced and also get your body to do the initiative for you.

The hardest part of this diet regimen is to discipline yourself to not consume at all times. We have been advised that we eat 5 or 6 meals a day (which is great if they're little dishes), yet this isn't the case for a great deal of people. With periodic fasting, you will be able to get the outcomes that you want without needing to work so hard.

Intermittent fasting is not simply a weight-loss diet strategy. It means far more than that. It

has some health and wellness benefits that will not just make you slimmer but much healthier as well as disease-free. If you are taking into consideration reduced carbohydrate, intermittent fasting can help you with that.

Low carbohydrate diet plans might suggest limiting carbs to 100 or perhaps 50 grams each day. This suggests cutting back on sugars, starches as well as all high carb foods. Obviously this is far better for your body, because your pancreas does not have to work as hard to eliminate sugars from you system.

Intermittent fasting recommends fasting for a figured out amount of time (whole lots of individuals fast for 24 hours, after that they consume healthy for the next 24 hours, and more). This shows your body needs to scavenge around for food (fuel), as well as does away with aged or broken cells and other waste that has accumulated in your body.

Incorporate the 2 of these for "Low Carb Intermittent Fasting," as well as you'll have a winning mix to going down weight as well as experience fantastic!

You should not eat foods for a 24-hour period when you are fasting. You can still have reduced carb and reduced calorie beverages such as water and also black coffee. You can eat healthy and balanced meals, but you must still watch your carbohydrate intake, outlook at labels, as well as research study foods to understand the finest options for your body as well as your health and wellness.

This is a way of life modification that should be a constant technique of consuming for you (a minimum of the low carbs). You need to make an effort to make healthy foods as well as drink options!

Incorporate low carb intermittent fasting together with workout. Soon, you will be in shape before you recognize it and will also feel fantastic.

Periodic fasting minimizes fat oxidation and also may decrease body weight. Exercising will certainly speed the process along and will certainly help you eliminate loose and flabby skin as well as get toned.

Intermittent fasting that has been performed on animals reveal a life-span increase of 40% or even more. That's amazing! This demonstrates exactly how much consuming healthy and balanced meals, and also cleansing your body can benefit not just your system and assist you lower weight, but also increase your days on this planet.

Reduced carbohydrate food choices are vegetables. You can consume as many vegetable as you want. Meats and also fish are fantastic dinner choices. For lunch you could make a salad with a boiled egg, onion and also a touch of cheese. Watch out for the carbs in the dressing nonetheless.

As long as you plan to eat healthy, your need for carbohydrates and sugars will possibly be gone. That need will definitely be decreased! You'll no longer want greasy, pleasant foods, when you start choosing to consume healthy and balanced, low carb foods.

And also keep in mind that prior to starting any kind of diet plan technique or workout routine, you need to constantly talk to your health care specialist! You want to make sure you stay healthy and balanced while getting much healthier!

Many thanks for reading this book. I hope it was practical and also provided you with every resources you need to meet your fitness goals.

The following activity is to start on your journey with intermittent fasting.

Intermittent fasting provides a great deal of benefits for your body. Whether you are aiming to reduce weight or improve your wellness, intermittent fasting is the way to go.

There are similarly a great deal of selections that come with periodic fasting so you can choose the option that will certainly function well for you. Periodic fasting is fundamental, simple to work with, and also effective. When you are ready to reduce weight or improve your health and wellness, revisit this guidebook to help you begin.